Drug Education Library

Diet Drugs

by Hal Marcovitz

LUCENT BOOKS
An imprint of Thomson Gale, a part of The Thomson Corporation

THOMSON
GALE™

Detroit • New York • San Francisco • San Diego • New Haven, Conn.
Waterville, Maine • London • Munich

THOMSON
GALE

Produced by OTTN Publishing, Stockton, N.J.

For more information, contact
Lucent Books
27500 Drake Rd.
Farmington Hills, MI 48331-3535
Or you can visit our Internet site at http://www.gale.com

LIBRARY OF CONGRESS CATALOGING-IN-PUBLICATION DATA

Marcovitz, Hal.
Diet drugs / by Hal Marcovitz.
p. cm. — (Drug education library)
Includes bibliographical references and index.
Summary: Discusses the history of diet drugs, use of diet drugs, fen-phen debacle, ephedra, diet drug use in weight loss, and the abuse of diet drugs.
ISBN 1-56006-914-7 (hard cover : alk. paper)
1. Diet drugs—Physiological effect—Juvenile literature. 2. Diet drug addiction—Health aspects—Juvenile literature. I. Title. II. Series.

Printed in China

CONTENTS

Foreword

The development of drugs and drug use in America is a cultural paradox. On the one hand, strong, potentially dangerous drugs provide people with relief from numerous physical and psychological ailments. Sedatives like Valium counter the effects of anxiety; steroids treat severe burns, anemia, and some forms of cancer; morphine provides quick pain relief. On the other hand, many drugs (sedatives, steroids, and morphine among them) are consistently misused or abused. Millions of Americans struggle each year with drug addictions that overpower their ability to think and act rationally. Researchers often link drug abuse to criminal activity, traffic accidents, domestic violence, and suicide.

These harmful effects seem obvious today. Newspaper articles, medical papers, and scientific studies have highlighted the myriad problems drugs and drug use can cause. Yet, there was a time when many of the drugs now known to be harmful were actually believed to be beneficial. Cocaine, for example, was once hailed as a great cure, used to treat everything from nausea and weakness to colds and asthma. Developed in Europe during the 1880s, cocaine spread quickly to the United States where manufacturers made it the primary ingredient in such everyday substances as cough medicines, lozenges, and tonics. Likewise, heroin, an opium derivative, became a popular painkiller during the late nineteenth century. Doctors and patients flocked to American drugstores to buy heroin, described as the optimal cure for even the worst coughs and chest pains.

As more people began using these drugs, though, doctors, legislators, and the public at large began to realize that they were more damaging than beneficial. After years of using heroin as a painkiller, for example, patients began asking their doctors for larger and stronger doses. Cocaine users reported dangerous side effects, including hallucinations and wild mood shifts. As a result, the U.S. government initiated more stringent regulation of many powerful and addictive drugs, and in some cases outlawed them entirely.

A drug's legal status is not always indicative of how dangerous it is, however. Some drugs known to have harmful effects can be purchased legally in the United States and elsewhere. Nicotine, a key ingredient in cigarettes, is known to be highly addictive. In an effort to meet their bodies' demands for nicotine, smokers expose themselves to lung cancer, emphysema, and other life-threatening conditions. Despite these risks, nicotine is legal almost everywhere.

Other drugs that cannot be purchased or sold legally are the subject of much debate regarding their effects on physical and mental health. Marijuana, sometimes described as a gateway drug that leads users to other drugs, cannot legally be used, grown, or sold in this country. However, some research suggests that marijuana is neither addictive nor a gateway drug and that it might actually benefit cancer and AIDS patients by reducing pain and encouraging failing appetites. Despite these findings and occasional legislative attempts to change the drug's status, marijuana remains illegal.

The Drug Education Library examines the paradox of drugs and drug use in America by focusing on some of the most commonly used and abused drugs or categories of drugs available today. By discussing objectively the many types of drugs, their intended purposes, their effects (both planned and unplanned), and the controversies surrounding them, the books in this series provide readers with an understanding of the complex role drugs and drug use play in American society. Informative sidebars, annotated bibliographies, and organizations to contact lists highlight the text and provide young readers with many opportunities for further discussion and research.

Diet Drugs: No Miracle Cures

Obesity has reached epidemic proportions in the United States today. According to the U.S. Centers for Disease Control and Prevention (CDC), nearly a third of all adults in the United States—more than 60 million people—are obese. The American Obesity Association estimates that nearly 10 million Americans between the ages of twelve and nineteen are overweight, while almost 5 million are obese. Today, people who are either overweight or obese make up about 64 percent of the U.S. population.

Being obese has been shown to lead to debilitating health consequences, such as heart disease, diabetes, and hypertension. The CDC estimates that almost 400,000 people die every year from diseases related to obesity.

To prevent potential health problems, many Americans have been taking steps to slim down. Across the country, health clubs are packed with people running on treadmills, lifting weights, swimming, and exercising in aerobics classes. Dieters are choosing from among hundreds of books by nutritional experts and physicians professing to know the best programs for keeping the weight off. And weight-watchers are selecting from the many low-calorie foods and diet beverages being offered on the shelves of their supermarkets. Some Americans, however, in search of a quick and easy method to slim down, are turning to another alternative: diet drugs.

An Array of Choices

The Center for Consumer Freedom estimates that Americans spend around $50 billion a year trying to lose weight. Much of that money goes to the diet drug industry, which produces both prescription and nonprescription weight-loss aids.

These weight-loss products can work in various ways. Some block the ability of the body to absorb fat. Others are stimulants that speed up the body's metabolic rate, while suppressing the appetite. Still others are diuretics, substances that decrease the amount of fluid in the body, resulting in water weight loss.

Some weight-loss drugs are sold only by prescription. Two of the most common ones used to treat obesity are orlistat (marketed by GlaxoSmithKline as Xenical) and sibutramine (sold by Abbott Laboratories as Meridia).

However, most weight-loss products can be bought without a prescription, or as over-the-counter (OTC) drugs. Many OTC weight-loss aids contain or consist of dietary supplements, so called because they are products taken by mouth and in addition to (or supplementing) a regular diet. Unlike synthetically made drugs, dietary supplements are substances found in nature, such as vitamins, minerals, amino acids, and plants.

Hundreds of weight-loss products are made with herbal or plant-based dietary supplements such as bitter orange, hoodia gordonii, and green tea extract. Sold in tablet, capsule, gel, liquid, and powder forms, these products can be easily purchased at supermarkets, pharmacies, health food stores, and on the Internet. According to the *Nutrition Business Journal*, over-the-counter weight-loss aids account for nearly $2 billion in sales each year in the United States.

Overweight or Obese?

Sales of diet drugs have remained strong as Americans continue to search for ways to lose unwanted fat. Most carry too much weight because they eat more food than their bodies can use.

Food and drink provide energy, measured in units called calories, that the human body burns as fuel. The average 150-pound person burns about 1,800 calories a day. Much more is used if the person engages in physical exercise. However, when a person consumes more calories than are burned, the leftovers are stored as fat. For every 3,500 extra calories consumed, the body adds about a pound. When too many pounds are gained, the person becomes overweight.

Physicians determine whether people are at healthy weight, overweight, or obese by using the "Body Mass Index," or BMI. The BMI is calculated by using a simple mathematical formula—dividing an individual's weight by the square of his or her height. An adult is considered overweight when the BMI ranges between 25.0 and 29.9, and obese when the BMI is 30 or greater. For example, a six-foot-tall man (1.8m) who weighs 162 pounds (73.5kg) has a BMI of 22, which is in the normal weight range. But a six-foot-tall man who weighs 192 pounds (87.1kg) has a BMI of 26, which is in the overweight range. And if that man weighs 258 pounds (117kg), he has a BMI of 35, which is in the obese range.

When a patient is identified as overweight, he or she will be advised to try to lose weight by eating a low-fat, low calorie diet; reducing food intake; and exercising regularly to burn off extra calories. If a person is obese, doctors often provide the same weight-loss program advice, but may also prescribe the use of diet drugs.

Some people have questioned whether it is appropriate to use drugs to treat obesity. They believe changes in eating and exercise habits can provide effective weight-loss results. However, in 1994, the Institute of Medicine, which is part of the National Academy of Sciences, suggested that obesity should not be regarded as a lifestyle choice. Instead, it should be viewed as a chronic condition—similar to high blood pressure, back pain, migraine headaches, or asthma. The institute recommended that doctors treat obese patients the same way they care for patients with chronic health problems, by including drug therapy as part of their treatment.

Prescription diet drugs have been proven to help obese patients lose weight, but these drugs do not provide a miracle cure. Studies have shown that after the dieters stop taking these drugs (and most are supposed to be taken for only short periods of time, such as three months), patients tend to regain lost weight. The greatest success in keeping weight off occurs when patients establish the habit of following a nutritious diet and regular exercise regimen while taking the prescribed drug.

Obesity affects more than one third of the adult population in the United States. Studies show that obese adults suffer from almost twice as many chronic health problems as those with normal weight.

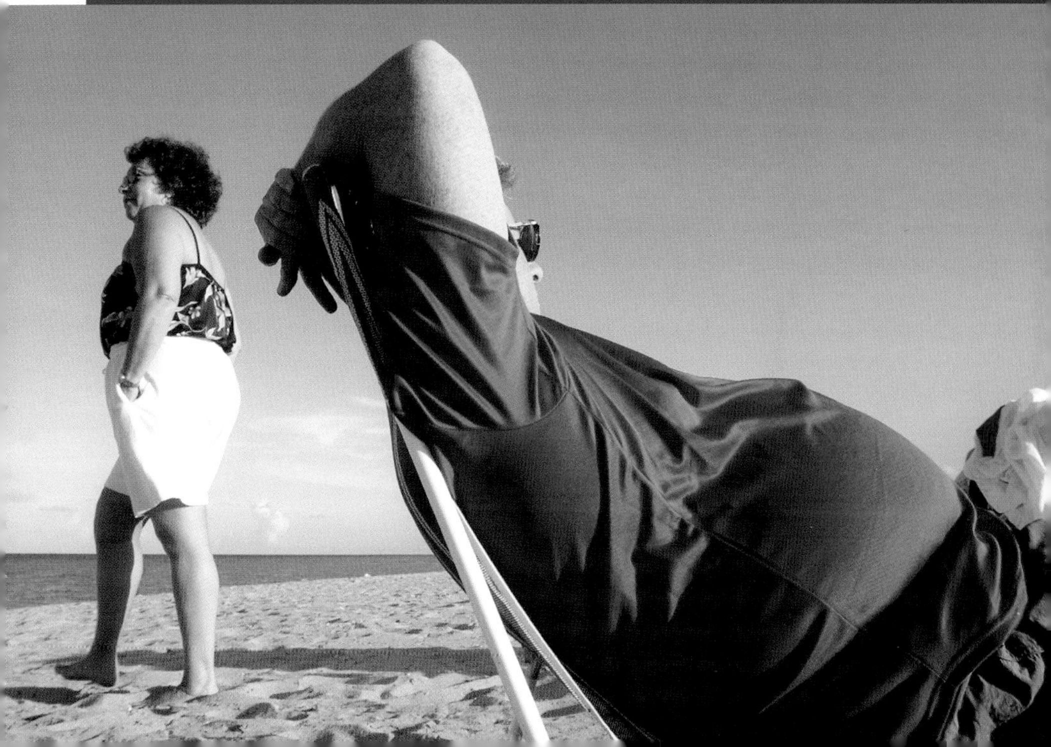

Calculating Body Mass Index (BMI)

BMI kg/m²	19	20	21	22	23	24	25	26	27	28	29	30	35	40	45
Height ft/in	Weight (lbs)														
4'10"	91	96	100	105	110	115	119	124	129	134	138	143	167	191	215
4'11'	94	99	104	109	114	119	124	128	133	138	143	148	173	198	222
5'	97	102	107	112	118	123	128	133	138	143	148	153	179	204	230
5'1"	100	106	111	116	122	127	132	137	143	148	153	158	185	211	238
5'2"	104	109	115	120	126	131	136	142	147	153	158	164	191	218	246
5'3"	107	113	118	124	130	135	141	146	152	158	163	169	197	225	254
5'4"	110	116	122	128	134	140	145	151	157	163	169	174	204	232	262
5'5"	114	120	126	132	138	144	150	156	162	168	174	180	210	240	270
5'6"	118	124	130	136	142	148	155	161	167	173	179	186	216	247	278
5'7"	121	127	134	140	146	153	159	166	172	178	185	191	223	255	287
5'8"	125	131	138	144	151	158	164	171	177	184	190	197	230	262	295
5'9"	128	135	142	149	155	162	169	176	182	189	196	203	236	270	304
5'10"	132	139	146	153	160	167	174	181	188	195	202	207	243	278	313
5'11"	136	143	150	157	165	172	179	186	193	200	208	215	250	286	322
6'	140	147	154	162	169	177	184	191	199	206	213	221	258	294	331
6'1"	144	151	159	166	174	182	189	197	204	212	219	227	265	302	340
6'2"	148	155	163	171	179	186	194	202	210	218	225	233	272	311	350
6'3"	152	160	168	176	184	192	200	208	216	224	232	240	279	319	359
6'4"	156	164	172	180	189	197	205	213	221	230	238	246	287	328	369
	Normal						Overweight					Obese		Extremely Obese	

Physicians use the Body Mass Index (BMI), a measure of the ratio of weight to height, to determine whether patients have a healthy weight or are considered overweight or obese.

The Dangers of Diet Drugs

Whenever someone takes a medication or dietary supplement, he or she runs the risk of experiencing adverse effects. The body may suffer a reaction to the drug or supplement, or the drug may interact dangerously with other drugs, supplements, or food that the person has consumed. Mild adverse reactions to diet drugs and weight-loss dietary supplements have included dizziness, headaches, nausea, and mood changes. More dangerous and even deadly reactions to these substances are increased blood pressure, heart attack, stroke, seizures, and kidney or liver failure.

Physicians know about possible adverse reactions for prescription drugs because these medicines must undergo rigorous testing and clinical trails before they can be marketed. Federal law requires their approval by the U.S. Food and Drug Administration (FDA), the federal agency in charge of evaluating the safety and effectiveness of drugs sold in the United States.

Ingredients common to many weight-loss supplements include ephedrine (or ephedra, from the herb Ma Huang), bitter orange, caffeine, and green tea extract.

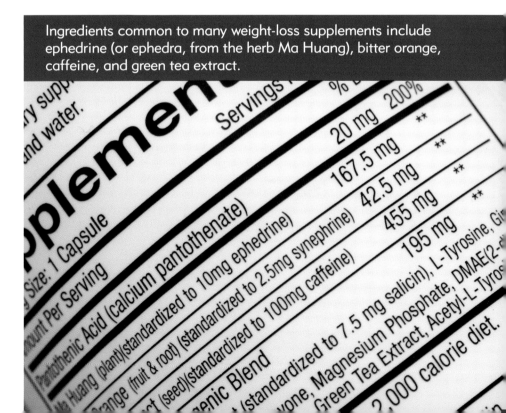

However, dietary supplements and supplement-based products do not have to be scientifically tested because they do not require FDA approval before being marketed and sold. Because little scientific research has been done on weight-loss dietary supplements, many physicians, nutritionists, and dieticians do not recommend their use. Many believe these products simply do not work and that they have not been proven to be safe.

In 2002, the U.S. Senate Committee on Governmental Affairs considered the issue of supplement safety at a hearing called "When Diets Turn Deadly: Consumer Safety and Weight-loss Supplements." The inquiry included testimony from Janet Heinrich, the director of public health issues for the U.S. Congress General Accounting Office. She testified about the growing popularity of weight-loss dietary supplements and warned about the dangers of using them:

> Obesity in the United States is reported to be a growing epidemic. And many more people are trying to lose weight. As sales of weight loss supplements have increased, so have concerns with their marketing and use. . . . For most weight loss supplements, there is little scientific evidence to support their efficacy. Although there have been studies on specific ingredients, many of these studies have been of short duration, involve small numbers of individuals or use study approaches that limited the usefulness of their findings.[1]

Over the years, news stories have linked serious health problems and even deaths to the use of diet drugs and weight-loss dietary supplements. Two of the most well publicized incidents involved the prescription drug fen-phen and the dietary supplement ephedra. Although there is growing awareness that diet drugs can be dangerous, people eager to find an easy way to lose weight continue to take them.

Chapter 1

A History of Dieting and Drug Use

The first diet drugs, which were sold in the United States during the latter part of the 1800s, had little scientific basis or proof that they worked. However, they sold widely because many people were willing to swallow just about anything advertised as guaranteed to help shed weight. For the most part, such "miracle cures" generally provided no benefit and sometimes caused more harm than good. Even when weight-loss drugs were developed later through legitimate scientific research, some were life-threatening and addictive.

No Need to Lose Weight

Throughout most human history, few people wanted to lose weight, because they had no extra weight to lose. For many centuries, most humans lived at the edge of starvation. For example, in Europe during the Middle Ages (A.D. 500 through 1500), the majority of people lived in extreme poverty, as village peasants, serfs laboring on their masters' lands, or beggars struggling to survive on city streets. These people considered themselves fortunate if they could find a few crumbs for their suppers.

During this time being plump was regarded as a desirable characteristic, an indicator of beauty and wealth. Obesity occurred mostly among the powerful—those who had access to unlimited food and drink. One of the most well-known was King Henry VIII, who ruled England during the sixteenth century. Henry, who became extremely obese in the latter years of his life, was said to have suffered from gout, commonly referred to at the time as the "disease of kings." Gout is an arthritic condition caused by the formation of uric acid crystals in the joints, particularly in the toes, resulting in extreme pain. Gout is often attributed to overindulgence in wine and sugar-rich foods—the type of diet that can cause significant weight gain. Because royalty could easily enjoy such diets, its members tended to suffer from gout more than the common people did.

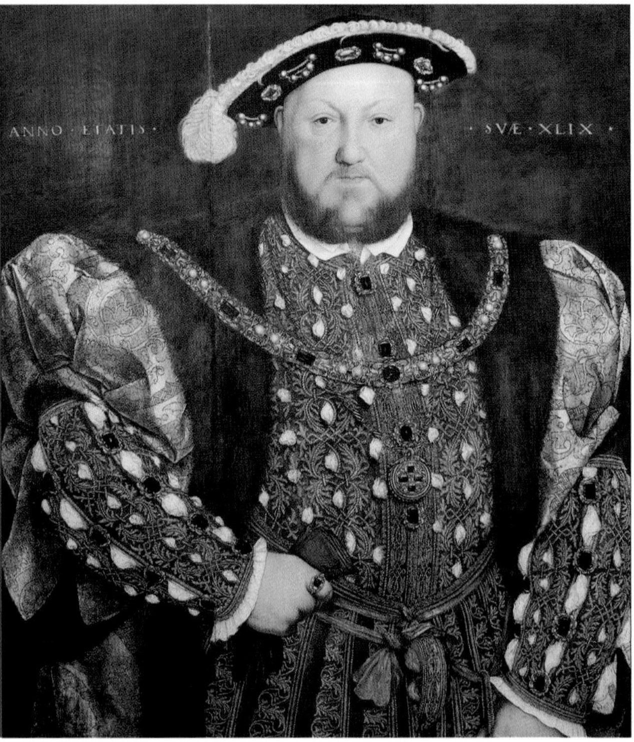

This portrait of King Henry VIII of England, painted by Hans Holbein the Younger in 1540, shows that the monarch became extremely obese in his later years. Being heavy was considered desirable during the sixteenth century, when only the privileged and wealthy had access to rich diets.

Overweight people did not understand that their obesity aggravated or caused health problems such as heart disease, backaches, shortness of breath, or gout. Being heavyset continued to be seen as a desirable characteristic for many centuries.

Overeating and Dieting

It was not until the mid-1800s that being fat became less of a status symbol in both the United States and Europe. People who were overweight turned to home remedies to shed pounds. Some cures bordered on the absurd. Writing in the 1847 medical journal *Primitive Physic*, a Dr. Scomberg recommended the following for a person who overeats: "If it be without vomiting, [the insatiable desire of eating] is often cured by a small bit of bread dipped in wine, and applied to the nostrils."[2]

In 1862, when a London undertaker named William Banting, who weighed more than 200 pounds (90.7 kilograms), decided he was too heavy, he followed his doctor's recommendation to eat only foods that did not contain sugar and starch. Scientists at the time did not fully understand the nutrients that made up food. Although bread contains starch, it was allowed in Banting's diet if it was toasted because people believed toasting reduced the starch content.

After following what essentially was a low-carbohydrate diet, Banting happily reported a weight loss of around 50 pounds (22.7 kg). In 1863, he shared his successful diet plan in a bestselling booklet entitled "Letter on Corpulence Addressed to the Public." This first diet book was so popular that several editions were published. People would ask each other whether they were on diets by saying, "Do you bant?"

In the mid-1800s few people were as heavy as Banting. However by the end of the century obesity was more common. People's lifestyles were changing dramatically because of the industrial revolution that had swept through Europe and United States. With the invention of power-driven machinery and the rise of factories, work became less labor-intensive and jobs became more sedentary. At the same time, food was becoming more plentiful and affordable for the growing middle class, and more and more fatty foods found their way into the everyday diet. As a result, more people became overweight.

Understanding Weight Gain

As people in the United States were putting on weight, doctors and scientists were trying to better understand what was in foods that made people fat. Beginning in the 1890s, chemist Wilbur Olin Atwater and physicist E. B. Rosa published several reports in which they described the energy content, measured in calories, of various foods. However, it was not until the following century that nutritionists used information about calories to develop weight-loss programs based on low-calorie diets.

Unaware of the importance of calories and diet, physicians in the mid 1890s looked for other causes of obesity. Some believed that the lack of the thyroid hormone caused people to become extremely overweight, and doctors began to prescribe animal-based thyroid pills to treat them. Other physicians were beginning to understand the connection between human nutrition and exercise.

One man who sought to educate the public about the importance of choosing nutritious food and following other health reforms was Dr. John Harvey Kellogg. Based in Battle Creek, Michigan, where he practiced as a surgeon, Kellogg published more than fifty books and pamphlets and ran a world-famous health clinic that supported his ideas on good health and fitness. Physical well-being occurred, he believed, when one ate a proper diet, exercised, and got adequate fresh air and rest.

Along with his brother, Will Keith Kellogg, John founded the Sanitas Food Company, which in 1897 began producing whole grain dry cereals so that Americans could easily eat a nutritious breakfast. However, a few years later the two dissolved their partnership, and in 1906 Will started his own business, which eventually became the Kellogg Company.

The Anti-Fat King

For a brief time, the Sanitas factory employed a man named Frank Jonas Kellogg, who was no relation to the founder. Frank Kellogg was born in Ohio and, after serving in the Civil War, moved to Battle Creek, where he found work as an artist, sign painter, and later a foreman in Kellogg's factory. Soon after leaving the cereal factory, Kellogg combined the well-known Kellogg name with the title of professor, and began creating and selling patent medicines.

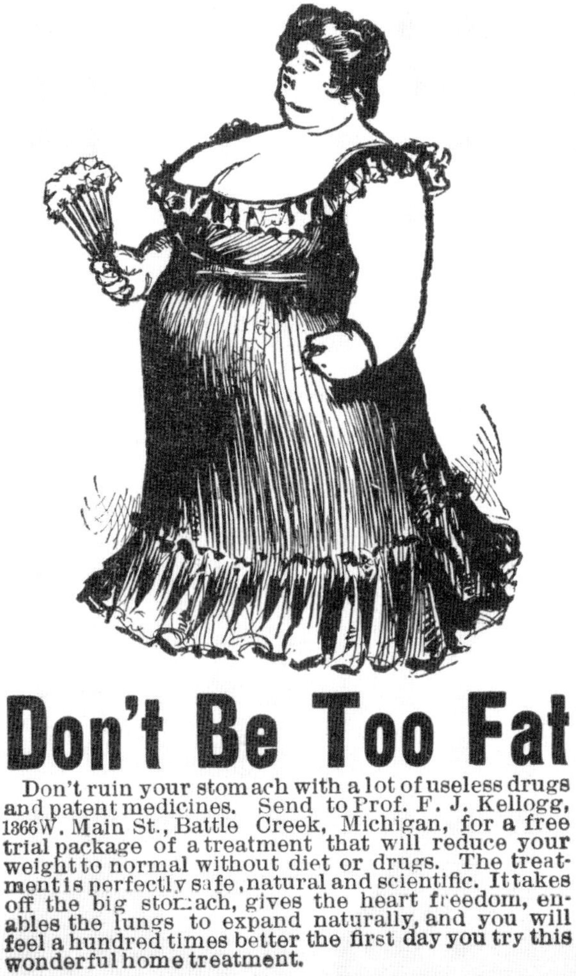
Don't Be Too Fat
Don't ruin your stomach with a lot of useless drugs and patent medicines. Send to Prof. F. J. Kellogg, 1366 W. Main St., Battle Creek, Michigan, for a free trial package of a treatment that will reduce your weight to normal without diet or drugs. The treatment is perfectly safe, natural and scientific. It takes off the big stomach, gives the heart freedom, enables the lungs to expand naturally, and you will feel a hundred times better the first day you try this wonderful home treatment.

Advertisement for "Professor" Frank J. Kellogg's weight-loss patent medicine. Many people confused the patent medicine manufacturer's questionable products with those of the real Dr. John Harvey Kellogg.

Some Unusual Dieting Tactics

Since the earliest times, dieting tactics have ranged from the absurd to the bizarre. In 1087, William the Conqueror found he was too heavy to climb atop his horse. In order to lose weight, he took to his bed for six months, refusing to eat or drink anything except alcoholic beverages. Although William managed to slim down, he died later that year when he fell off his horse.

During the early twentieth century, some diets of questionable nutritional value found fervent followers in the United States. One popular 1905 fad promoted the idea that smoking cigarettes suppressed the desire for sugar. In 1932, beauty parlors offered Dr. Stoll's Slimming Powder, a product composed of milk chocolate, whole wheat, and other starchy ingredients—hardly the ingredients one would expect to find in the diet of someone trying to lose weight.

Author Robert Linn promoted a highly unusual diet in his 1976 book *The Last Chance Diet*. In it, he urged people to eat no food at all, and instead to live entirely on a drink called Prolinn. He developed this liquid protein out of slaughterhouse byproducts such as horns, tendons, bones, hooves, and hides that had been ground up and treated with enzymes.

Patent medicines were products made by mixing various substances into elixirs that promised to cure specific ailments. The name originated in seventeenth-century England, where the first concoctions were sold under royal endorsement, or "patent." Often derided as quacks and charlatans, the makers of patent medicines were known to create "cures" that seldom actually worked.

"Professor" Kellogg became the first in the patent medicine industry to specialize in the diet pill business. He declared himself the Anti-Fat King, and in 1893 began selling tablets that promised to strip the fat from a person's body. Within ten years he was marketing a variety of similar products with such names as Rengo, Malto-Fructo, Sanitone Wafers, Frank J. Kellogg's Safe Fat Reducer, and Professor Kellogg's Brown Tablets. His diet pills, which seemed to work, were an immediate hit. Their sales made him into a millionaire practically overnight.

However, Kellogg soon attracted the attention of the American Medical Association (AMA), which had started lobbying the federal government demanding regulation of the patent medicine industry. AMA doctors analyzed some of Kellogg's concoctions and declared them to be nothing more than a mixture of thyroid extract, various herbs, seeds, and even toasted bread. Some of the ingredients, the doctors pointed out, provided a laxative effect, which could explain why Kellogg's customers believed they were losing weight. But when taken at the doses Professor Kellogg recommended, the products, because of their thyroid content, could cause dangerous effects such as hypertension, cardiac arrest, or stroke.

Rather than fight the AMA, Kellogg simply removed the thyroid extract from his original recipe and went into the business of selling laxatives. After his death in 1916, his heirs stayed in the laxative business until 1940, when dwindling sales forced them to fold the company.

Opium, Herbs, and Tapeworms

Even though Kellogg left the diet pill business, other patent medicine makers continued to provide obesity remedies. Because the patent medicine industry in the United States was virtually unregulated, there were hundreds of so-called miracle drugs that claimed to cure illnesses ranging from sore throats to diarrhea to baldness. Most patent medicines consisted of common herbs and spices, although they were often laced with opium, a narcotic drug that dulls the senses and induces sleep.

The addictive qualities of opium were not known until 1914, when it was outlawed in the United States. Until then it was a common patent medicine ingredient. A mother who gave her toddler a dose of Mrs. Winslow's Soothing Syrup to ease the pain of teething was actually unknowingly treating her child with a dangerous narcotic.

Patent medicine manufacturers often advertised in newspapers and magazines. For example, in the late 1890s, Dr. Edison's Obesity Remedies proclaimed its product had cured local socialite Mary Manning by melting 35 pounds (15.8kg) off her frame. She even included her own letter of recommendation in the ad, which stated:

> Mary Hyde Manning, one of the best known of Troy's, New York, society women, grew too fleshy, and used Dr. Edison's Obesity Remedies. Read the letter telling of her reduction and restoration to health: —"In six weeks I was reduced 35 pounds, from 171 to 136, by Dr. Edison's Obesity Pills and Reducing Tablets. I recommend these remedies to all fat and sick men and women."[3]

Another patent medicine, Warner's Obesity Tablets promised an "effective cure for gradually reducing obesity and over fatness."[4]

Manufacturers of patent medicines seldom provided information in their advertisements about the content of their products, although one ad for Warner's Obesity Tablets claimed that the pills would turn tap water into high quality mineral water. In other words, the ad implied, the tablets contained minerals.

Some patent medicine manufacturers advertised that their obesity pills contained the heads of tapeworms—parasites that can live in uncooked meats and fish and that spread in places when sanitation is inadequate. Weight loss would

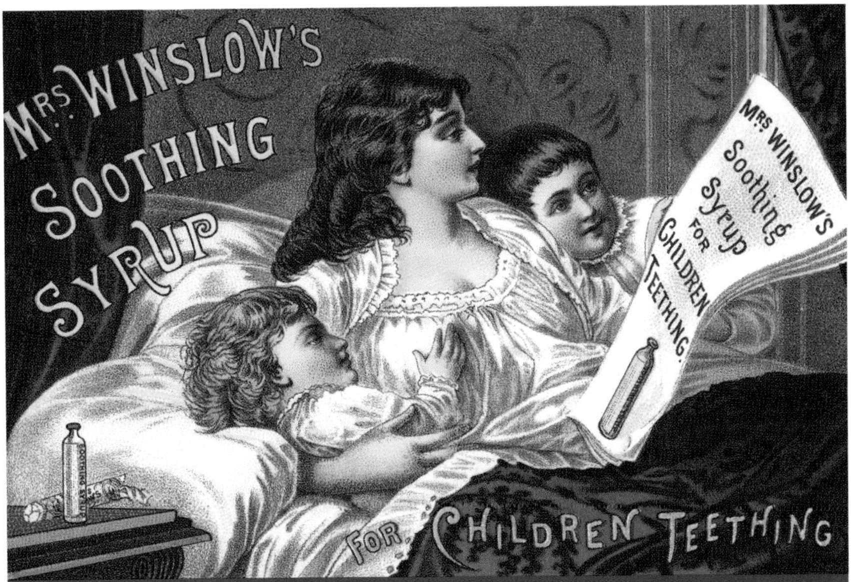

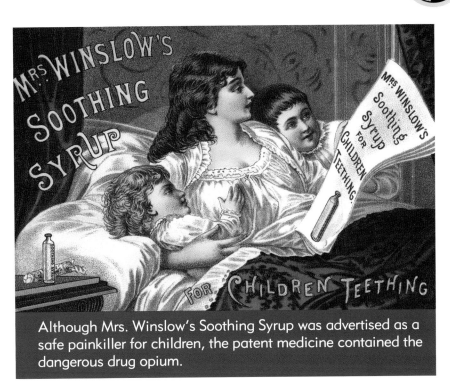

Although Mrs. Winslow's Soothing Syrup was advertised as a safe painkiller for children, the patent medicine contained the dangerous drug opium.

occur with their products, these pill makers claimed, because the tapeworm would grow inside the stomach and absorb food eaten by the host. No one knows whether such pills actually contained tapeworm heads, although it is likely they did not. (If someone did swallow a tapeworm, the result would hardly be a svelte figure. A person with a tapeworm infection would suffer nausea, weakness, loss of appetite, diarrhea, and abdominal pain; however, he or she would not lose weight.)

Before 1906, manufacturers of patent medicines did not have to inform consumers about the ingredients used in their products. That year the U.S. Congress passed the U.S. Pure Food and Drug Act, which required drug makers to disclose ingredients on the labels. These requirements proved too stringent for the patent medicine companies, and they were soon driven out of business.

Maria Callas and the Iodine Diet

For much of her life, Greek opera star Maria Callas (1923–1977) battled weight problems. At one point during her career, she weighed 237 pounds (108kg). In 1954, when opera director Luchino Visconti told Callas he would not work with her unless she lost weight, Callas quickly shed 105 pounds (48kg). Many people wondered how the singer had lost so much weight so quickly. The answer remained a mystery until 2005, when the *London Observer* reported that Callas lost the weight by consuming a diet based on iodine.

The chemical element iodine makes the thyroid gland more active. Located beneath the larynx, the thyroid helps regulate growth and metabolism. If the gland is sluggish—a condition known as hypothyroidism—the reduced amount of iodine in the body can cause impotence, irritability and forgetfulness, and weight gain.

Too much iodine can cause skin irritations, stomach pain, fever, nausea, inability to urinate, thirst and vomiting. Bruno Tosi, president of the Maria Callas Association, told the *Observer* that the singer's iodine treatments caused her to suffer many side effects. However, he said, they helped her turn into "a beautiful swan."

Quoted in Barbara McMahon, "Revealed: Callas's Secret Passion for Recipes She Refused to Taste," *London Observer*, July 24, 2005. www.guardian.co.uk/italy/story/0,12576,1535128,00.html.

A New Diet Drug

Products that originated in chemical laboratories soon replaced the potions that had been marketed as patent medicines. One major ingredient for what would become a common weight-loss drug had been discovered in the 1880s, when a Japanese chemist named Nagayoshi Nagai extracted the active ingredient ephedrine from the ephedra plant. Within a few years, researchers learned that ephedrine could be used to treat asthma, because it helped open up clogged bronchial passages. In 1887 a German chemist named L. Edeleano combined ephedrine with other chemicals, synthesizing a drug that became known as amphetamine. The drug, which he called phenylisopropylamine, was initially used to treat people with chest and nasal congestion. However, drug makers soon discovered that amphetamines could be used for many other purposes, including helping people lose weight.

In 1927, researchers classified amphetamine as a stimulant because of its effect on the central nervous system. Amphetamines stimulate the nervous system, raising blood pressure, accelerating the heart rate, constricting blood vessels, and causing sweating. Because amphetamines speed up the basal metabolic rate—the rate the body burns energy while at rest—the drug can aid weight loss. Researchers also found that amphetamines suppress appetite, so that people taking the drugs consume fewer calories throughout the day.

Growing Amphetamine Use

Around the 1930s physicians began prescribing amphetamines as diet pills. Over the next three decades, people trying to lose weight took millions of doses of amphetamines in the United States.

Amphetamines grew in popularity in many other parts of the world as well. In Sweden, researchers estimated in 1942 that about 3 percent of the population was taking amphetamines regularly. Millions more consumed them occasionally. Most Swedes did not take the drugs in an effort to lose weight; rather, they took amphetamines because of another effect of the drug: it elevates mood and makes people feel good.

Soon, it became clear that amphetamine users were becoming dependent on the drug, which has strong addictive qualities. It also caused serious side effects. Long-term amphetamine users suffered from disrupted sleep, depression, fatigue, irrational behavior, hallucinations, delusions, and even brain damage. Concerned about the growing numbers of people becoming addicted to amphetamines, the Swedish government took steps in 1944 to strictly control the drug's distribution in the country.

In response, a black market (the illegal trade) of the drug evolved, as Swedes smuggled large quantities of American-made diet pills into the country. Some were derivatives of amphetamines, such as dextroamphetamine (marketed as Dexedrine) and methamphetamine (Desoxyn). Swedish authorities struggled to keep American-made diet pills from entering their country. In a 1968 study, college professor Gunnar Inghe wrote of the growing problem in Sweden:

> Recent reports tell of an increasing abuse of weight-reducing preparations. . . . The misusers themselves have an incredible capacity for rapidly progressing to new euphoria-inducing preparations, which apparently without exception can prove both habit-forming and dependence-forming.[5]

Amphetamine Abuse

People also abused amphetamines in the United States. Truck drivers and students were known to take them as pep pills, because the drugs helped them stay awake and have more energy. During the 1950s and 1960s, abuse of prescription diet pills such as Benzedrine (amphetamine sulfate) and Dexedrine became widespread. The late country and western singer Johnny Cash admitted to developing an addiction to the diet drug Dexamyl (dextroamphetamine sulphate), while spending months on tour in the 1950s.

Because amphetamines enhance energy, professional athletes used them just before a game or competition. In his 1970 memoir, *Ball Four*, baseball pitcher Jim Bouton reported that Dexamyl was widely used throughout the Major

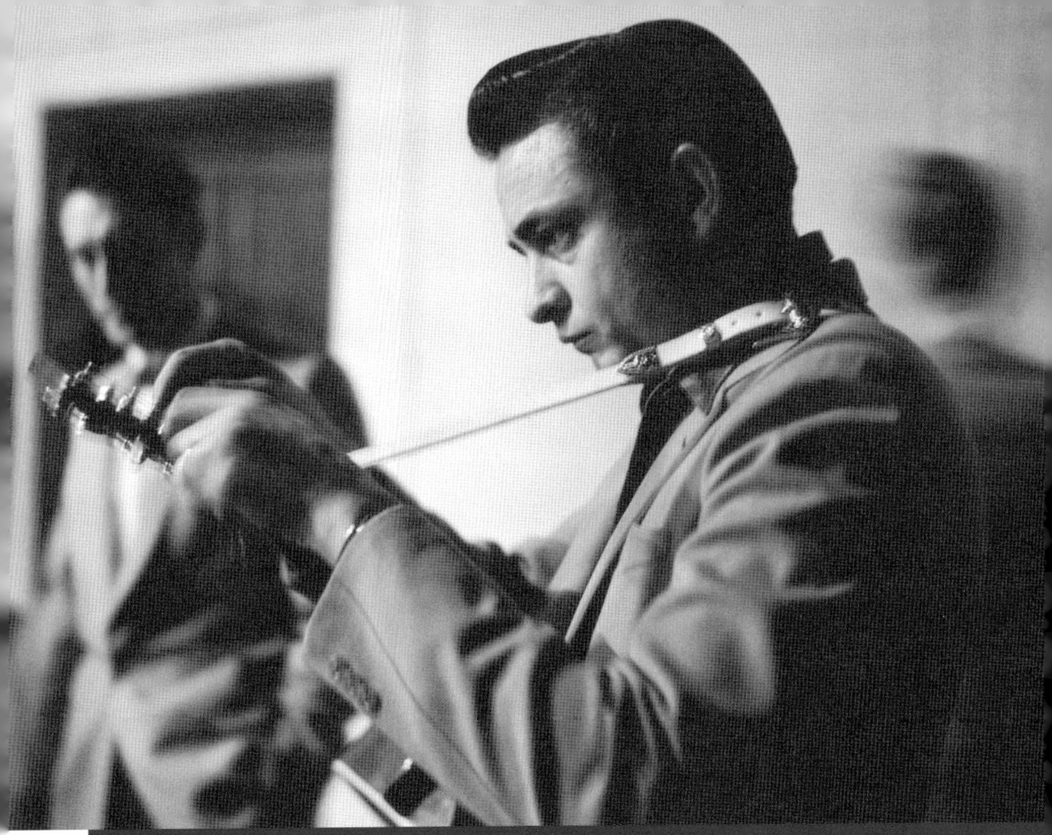

During the 1950s, singer Johnny Cash became addicted to amphetamines. He was even arrested in 1965 for smuggling the drug across the Mexican border inside his guitar case.

Leagues. In his book, Bouton explained that people referred to the green and white capsules as "greenies." And he and his fellow players were big fans. "Greenies are pep pills—dextroamphetamine sulphate—and a lot of baseball players couldn't function without them,"[6] Bouton reported.

Bouton also explained how easy it was for him and his teammates to obtain the prescription drugs:

> We've been running short of greenies. We don't get them from the trainer, because greenies are against club policy. So we get them from players on other teams who have friends who are doctors, or friends who know where to get greenies. One of our lads is going to have a bunch of greenies mailed to him by some of the guys on the Red Sox. And to think you can spend five years in jail for giving your friend a marijuana cigarette.[7]

After the addictive qualities of amphetamines were recognized, the U.S. government moved in the early 1970s to have access to them severely restricted. Because of their high potential for abuse and addiction, but their accepted use as treatment for certain medical conditions, amphetamines are classified as Schedule II drugs, as defined by the Controlled Substances Act. This law was passed by Congress in 1970 as part of the Comprehensive Drug Abuse Prevention and Control Act.

Although the legislation led to a decline in the use of amphetamines, some doctors continued to prescribe the drugs to help patients lose weight. In a speech published in the *Los Angeles Times*, herbal diet guru Mark Reynolds Hughes recalled how his mother became addicted to the amphetamine-based drug Dexamyl during the mid-1970s:

> My mom was always going out and trying some kind of funny fad diet as I was growing up. Eventually, she went to the doctor to get some help, and he prescribed to her Dexamyl, kind of a fad diet then. For those of you who don't know about it, it's a drug, a narcotic. It's a form of speed, or amphetamine. You're not able to eat or sleep. . . .
>
> After several years of using it, she ended up having to eat sleeping pills for her to sleep at night. And after several years of doing that, her body basically started to deteriorate. And she started seeing four or five doctors to keep her habit up.[8]

Because of the addictive qualities of amphetamines and their adverse effects (which include rapid heartbeat, erratic mood swings, and dangerously high blood pressure), physicians today do not prescribe their use as diet drugs. However, they continue to be available by prescription in the United States for the treatment of other health problems. The illegal use of amphetamines continues to be a public health concern.

Chapter 2

The Fen-Phen Debacle

As the dangers of amphetamine use became apparent during the 1960s and 1970s, the makers of diet drugs turned to other substances as ingredients for their weight-loss products. Some scientists discovered drugs that were in the same chemical class as amphetamines but did not have the same addictive qualities or stimulating effects. These new drugs helped create a new generation of diet drugs that worked, like amphetamines, as appetite suppressants—people who took the pills did not feel hungry.

Suppressing the Appetite with Serotonin

Drugs that eliminate hunger pains in the body work by affecting messages sent to the brain. The human brain consists of millions of neurons, which are the basic cells of the nervous system. Each neuron emits electrical impulses containing messages that control the body's functions. The impulses that pass through the body's network of nerve cells tell a foot to take a step, or a hand to hold a pencil, or the lips to form words so that the person may speak. Chemicals known as

Synaptic Transmission

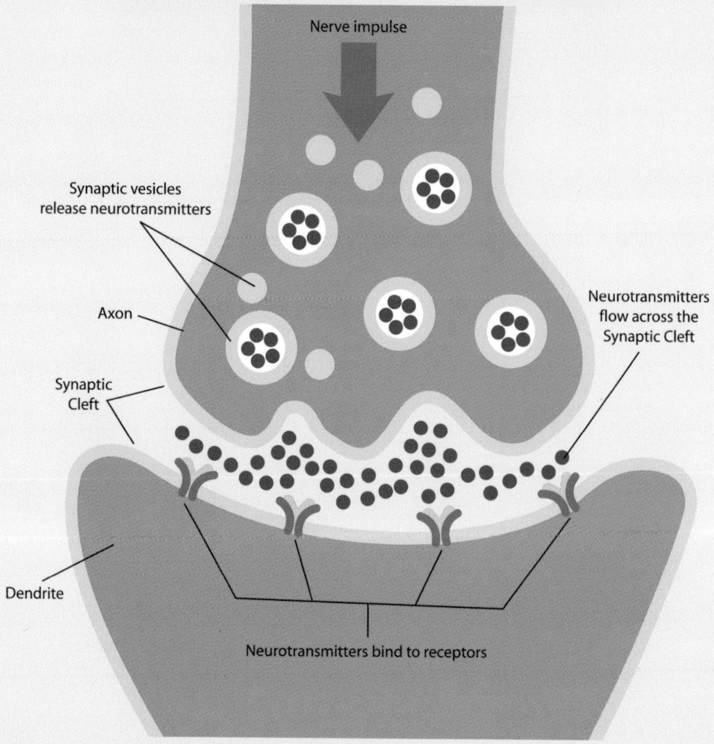

Neurons process and carry messages from the body to the brain and central nervous system. These messages, or impulses, must be transmitted across gaps between the neurons (synapses). Chemicals called neurotransmitters, which are released from synaptic vesicles in the axon of a nerve cell, carry the impulse across the synapse, and bind with receptors in the dendrite of an adjacent neuron. This enables the impuse to quickly move through the nervous system. Some diet drugs work by stimulating the release of the neurotransmitters serotonin and norepinephrine, which carry messages about appetite, hunger, and digestion to the brain.

neurotransmitters carry the messages from one neuron to another that tell the body what to do.

Certain neurotransmitters carry messages to the hypothalamus, the area of the brain that regulates appetite, hunger, and digestion. Located deep inside the brain and no larger than a walnut, the hypothalamus also controls body temperature, sleep, moods, and sex drive.

Some drugs can stimulate or block the neurotransmitters that affect the hypothalamus, with the result that the body does not feel hunger. In the early 1970s, Dr. Richard Wurtman, a neurologist at the Massachusetts Institute of Technology (MIT) suggested that a drug that could enhance the release of a neurotransmitter called serotonin (which reduces the desire to eat) might help deaden the urge to overeat.

Serotonin improves mood and provides an emotional feeling of satisfaction—of having had enough. The neurotransmitter also affects the gastrointestinal tract by slowing down digestion. When the body receives a serotonin rush to the hypothalamus, the digestive process slows and food remains in the stomach longer. As a result, the increase of serotonin suppresses the appetite by reducing the urge to eat as often.

Wurtman found that there is a relationship in the body between serotonin levels and appetite. After his research showed that carbohydrate intake helps elevate levels of serotonin, he theorized that many obese people ate and actually became addicted to carbohydrate-rich foods such as ice cream, French fries, cookies, and potato chips because such foods increased the serotonin levels in the body. The elevated serotonin levels elevated their mood. "We reasoned that people were using these foods as drugs,"[9] Wurtman stated. And they had become obese because of their addiction to them.

A Winning Combination

To help obese patients lose weight, Wurtman decided to use drugs, rather than food, to elevate serotonin levels in the body. In the early 1970s there were several drugs known to affect neurotransmitter levels in the body. Psychiatrists commonly used them in treating patients with mental illnesses, such as depression and paranoia.

Wurtman studied fenfluramine, a serotonin-enhancing drug manufactured by the French pharmaceutical maker Laboratoires Servier SA. He found that the drug reduced the appetite of obese patients. Patients taking the drug ate fewer snacks between meals, and felt full longer. "We tested [fenfluramine]," he told *Time*, "and we found that it worked in selectively suppressing carbohydrate overeating."[10]

In 1973, the Food and Drug Administration approved fenfluramine for use as a diet drug, and it was marketed in the United States by the pharmaceutical manufacturer American Home Products, under the name Pondimin. However, few physicians prescribed fenfluramine for their obese patients, mostly because the drug made its users drowsy.

The FDA had approved another weight-loss drug many years earlier, in 1959. Called phentermine, the drug stimulates the release of the neurotransmitter norepinephrine (which increases feelings of hunger). Although it would seem that increasing the flow of norepinephrine to the brain would increase feelings of hunger, that is not necessarily true. In fact, it has been shown that when phentermine or a similar drug is used to create a rush of norepinephrine, the body responds by feeling a decrease in appetite. Phentermine is a stimulant, and in the same drug class as amphetamine.

The Fen-Phen Study

In 1983, University of Rochester pharmacology professor Michael Weintraub theorized that an effective weight-loss drug could be obtained by combining phentermine and fenfluramine. The two drugs would enhance the release of the neurotransmitters serotonin and norepinephrine, which had been shown to suppress the appetite. In addition, the stimulating qualities of phentermine would counter the sleep-inducing side effect of fenfluramine.

A pharmacist holds the diet drugs Pondimin (fenfluramine) and Redux (dexfenfluramine). Redux contained fenfluramine and phentermine, or fen-phen, a drug combination that first became popular with dieters in 1992. The FDA approved the sale of Redux—a single pill containing both drugs—in 1996.

To test his theory, Weintraub administered doses of both fenfluramine and phentermine (or fen-phen) to 121 obese patients over a four-year period. The participants in the study were mostly women with an average weight of more than 200 pounds (90.7kg). During the course of the study, most of the patients lost an average of 32 pounds (14.5kg)—a much better result than that achieved when phentermine and fenfluramine were administered individually.

Weintraub published the results of his fen-phen study in 1992 in the *Journal of Clinical Pharmacology and Therapeutics.* The response was immediate. Because the study appeared to prove that the drug combination was so effective, physicians at weight-loss clinics rushed to provide their patients with prescriptions. However, because the fen-phen combination drug did not have FDA approval, doctors wrote prescriptions for it "off-label." That is, they wrote individual prescriptions for the two different diet drugs, and instructed their patients to take the drugs at the same time.

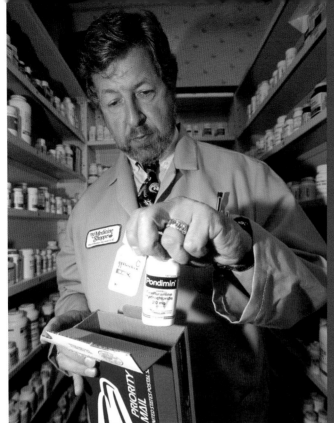

Obese patients who took the drug combination initially praised it, claiming that it helped them shed dozens of pounds. In 1995, Howard Hutson, a patient at a weight-loss clinic in Monsey, New York, told a reporter for *Fortune* magazine that when he first started taking fen-phen he weighed 450 pounds (204.1kg). The drug combination helped him shed 69 pounds (31.3kg), and he planned to continue taking it in hopes of losing another 150 pounds (68kg). "My main problem was always snacking and watching TV," Hutson told *Fortune*. "Now I've started to push food away before finishing it."[11]

The following year, the FDA granted approval for the sale of a combination fen-phen pill (called dexfenfluramine) to Interneuron, which owned U.S. rights to the drug. Subsequently, American Home Products bought the rights to market fen-phen, and its subsidiary Wyeth-Ayerst began selling dexfenfluramine under the name Redux.

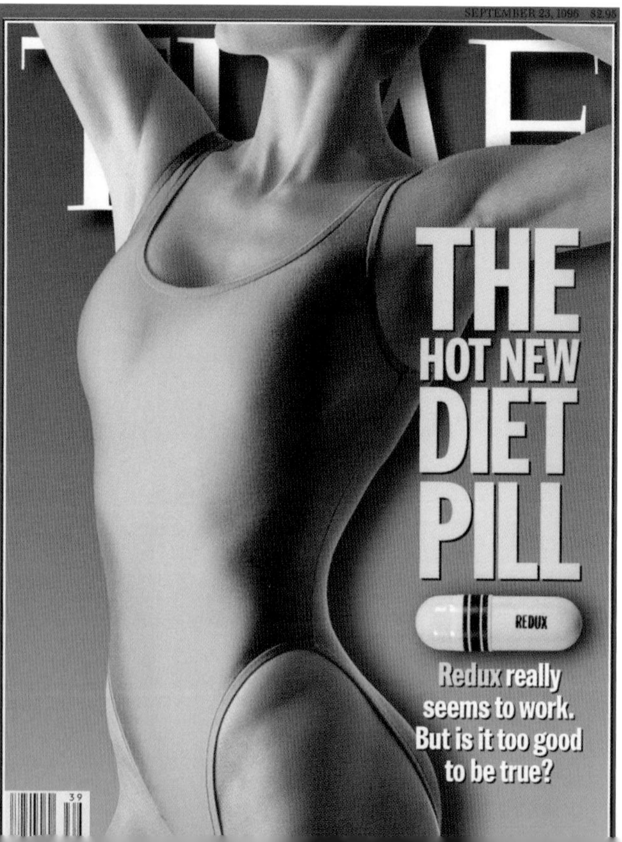

SEPTEMBER 23, 1996 $2.95
THE
HOT NEW
DIET
PILL
REDUX
Redux really seems to work. But is it too good to be true?

The September 23,1996, cover of *Time* magazine features the new diet pill Redux, or fen-phen. At the time this story appeared, reports of serious adverse effects caused by the drug had already surfaced.

Some doctors protested against the FDA approval. Critics argued that the health effects of the fen-phen combination had not been fully explored; some cited research that showed fen-phen had caused brain damage in mice and other animals. These physicians called on the FDA to withhold approval of the drug until further studies were conducted.

However, the fen-phen critics were overruled by FDA officials, who pointed out that approximately 10 million patients in Europe had been taking dexfenfluramine since the early 1980s, when Servier first produced the drug combination. Dr. James Bilstad, who served on an FDA panel that approved Redux, told *Time* magazine, "It is highly unlikely that there is anything significant in toxicity to the drug that hasn't been picked up with this kind of [widespread use]."[12]

The FDA approved Redux as a short-term (three-month) drug for the treatment of obesity. However, many people who were simply overweight also wanted to use the drug. In the United States alone, 2 million prescriptions were written for Redux during its first year on the market. Another 18 million prescriptions for fenfluramine and phentermine were written off-label, with instructions that they be taken in combination. Most fen-phen users were women in their thirties and forties who, after struggling with obesity for most of their lives, believed they had finally found a miracle cure.

Primary Pulmonary Hypertension

Although Redux users reported significant weight loss, many also noted unpleasant side effects as well. Soon after taking the drug, Redux patient Betty Moore experienced dramatic mood swings, she reported. "I kind of knew it had something to do with the medication," she said, "Because a couple of times when I went off it for a few days, it was almost like going off amphetamines."[13] (Symptoms of amphetamine withdrawal can include anxiety, insomnia, or depression.) Redux users also reported side effects such as headaches, diarrhea, dry mouth, and even drowsiness.

News of a very serious adverse effect linked to fen-phen use appeared in August 1996. Doctors reported in the *New England Journal of Medicine* that patients on fen-phen showed a greatly increased risk of developing primary pulmonary hypertension, or PPH. This rare, often fatal, lung disease is due to an abnormal thickening of the walls of the pulmonary artery—the blood vessel that carries blood from the heart to the lungs. The thickened blood vessel walls cause high blood pressure, or hypertension, in the pulmonary artery. Patients with primary pulmonary hypertension suffer from fatigue, dizziness, and shortness of breath with minimal exertion.

There is no cure for PPH, although patients may live for many years with the disease. Most pulmonary hypertension patients have to take blood-thinning drugs known as anticoagulants, which help to increase blood flow to the heart. As the disease progresses, it causes a decrease in the amount of oxygen present in the arterial blood. To survive, PPH patients need extra oxygen supplied by an oxygen tank. Some pulmonary hypertension patients must undergo lung transplants—radical surgery that is conducted in the most severe cases only.

Outrage, Shock, and Despair

In the television documentary *Dangerous Prescription*, a reporter from the PBS public affairs program *Frontline* interviewed Dr. Stuart Rich, one of the authors of the *New England Journal of Medicine* article. When asked to describe what he felt upon identifying the connection between PPH and fen-phen use, he replied:

> Do you want the truth? It was despair. My reaction was despair. Why despair? My specialty is—I treat patients with pulmonary hypertension. These are the sickest cardiovascular patients that exist. They're young people. They're tragic stories.
>
> We have some treatments—they are very difficult treatments. [PPH is] a death sentence, and it's a slow

> death, like drowning over months to years, if you can envision what that's like. My heart breaks with every new patient that's referred to me. . . . I'm now thinking that I'm going to go from 200 patients a year to 2,000 patients a year, and I despair. I'm not going to be able personally to deal with this epidemic of this horrible disease that I absolutely knew was coming around the corner because of this.
>
> Outrage, shock—you can name all those emotions. Despair. I was distraught over the notion of what's going to happen as a result of this.[14]

In the journal article the medical researchers estimated that a person who did not take fen-phen had a one or two in a million chance of contracting PPH. Those who took the diet drug combination, however, had increased their odds of developing the disease to forty-six in a million. Upon receiving news of the PPH link in patients taking fen-phen, Wyeth-

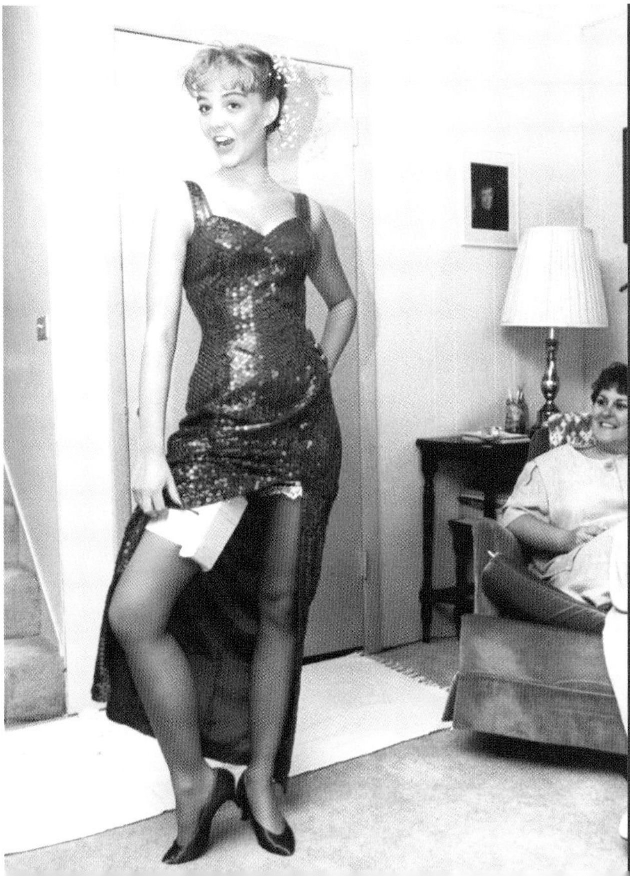

In August 1996, a study in the *New England Journal of Medicine* reported that fen-phen use could cause primary pulmonary hypertension, or PPH. Here, a victim of the deadly disease shows a battery-powered pump she must wear. The pump continuously administers the medicine she requires.

Ayerst changed the warning label on Redux to acknowledge the possibility of this adverse effect.

Valvular Heart Disease

But then another serious adverse effect linked to fen-phen use was reported in 1997. The Mayo Clinic of Rochester, Minnesota, informed the Food and Drug Administration that valvular heart disease had occurred in twenty-four of its patients who had been taking fen-phen. Several other medical

Heart Valve Damage

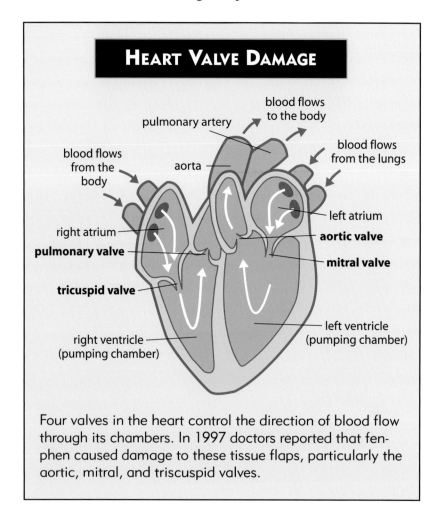

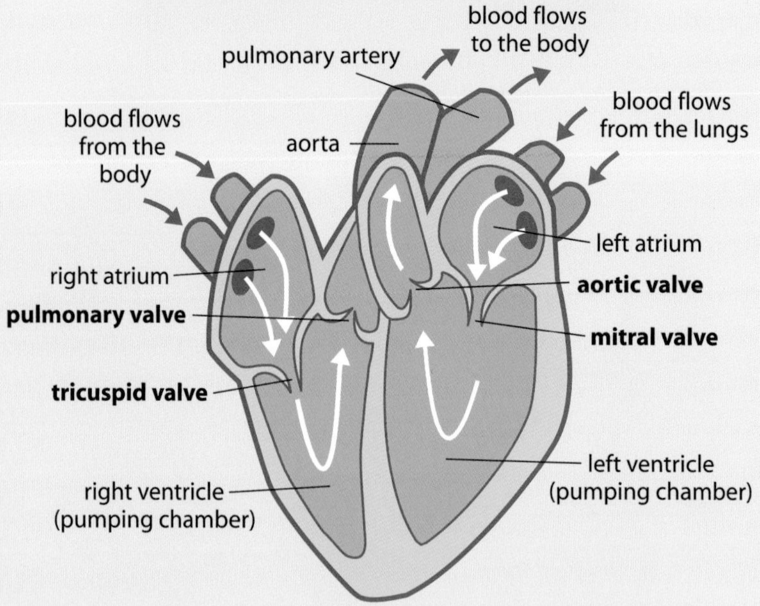

Four valves in the heart control the direction of blood flow through its chambers. In 1997 doctors reported that fen-phen caused damage to these tissue flaps, particularly the aortic, mitral, and triscuspid valves.

institutions soon reported similar findings: heart damage had occurred in another 291 patients, most of them women, who had been taking the drug combination.

Eventually, medical researchers concluded that fen-phen caused valvular heart disease, a condition in which the heart valves become short, thick, and stiff and unable to properly close. The damaged heart valves allow some of the blood being pumped from the heart to leak back in. As a result, the heart is forced to pump harder than normal. Symptoms of valvular heart disease include shortness of breath, fatigue, rapid heartbeat, chest discomfort, and fainting spells. The condition can be fatal, and in many cases requires valve-replacement surgery or even a complete heart transplant.

Medical researchers predicted that 25 to 30 percent of people who had used fen-phen were likely to develop some degree of valvular heart disease. However, Mayo Clinic physician Donald Hensrud noted that it could be years before the disease starts showing up in former fen-phen users. "We may suddenly see a surge in valve disease among women, I guess, like an epidemic," he said. "We don't know, but we should be prepared for it."[15]

In September 1997, the FDA called on American Home Products to withdraw fenfluramine (Pondimin) and dexflenfluramine (Redux) from the market. Studies had shown that the drug phentermine, by itself, was not hazardous, and the federal agency allowed it to remain available to dieters for short-term use.

Massive Litigation

Some researchers estimate that as many as 6 million people in the United States took fen-phen before the drug was taken off the market. Many former fen-phen users and their relatives decided to sue the drug manufacturer because of their own health problems or deaths of loved ones.

In August 2000 American Home Products set up a $3.75 billion trust fund as part of an agreement to settle claims

Phen-Pro

When fenfluramine was taken off the market in 1997, doctors continued to write prescriptions for phentermine, which by itself had been used as a weight-loss drug with no harmful health effects. Because the antidepressant Prozac was also being successfully used as a diet drug, some doctors decided to combine the two drugs, creating a new diet drug known as phen-pro.

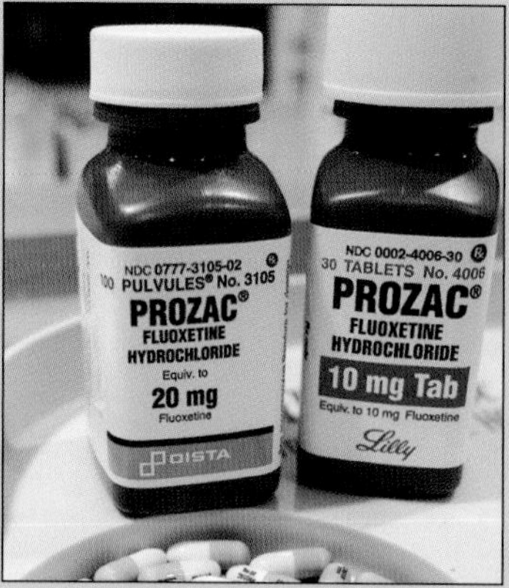

Prozac (fluoxetine) has been prescribed as a diet drug because it suppresses the appetite

The Food and Drug Administration has not approved this new drug combination, so doctors must write prescriptions off-label—providing two separate prescriptions for the drugs, with instructions to patients to take them together. Although patients have seen weight-loss results, some physicians disagree with this practice of writing diet drug prescriptions off-label. They point to the case of fen-phen, which was prescribed off-label for years, and subsequently linked to potentially fatal conditions affecting the heart and lungs. One dissenter is Georgetown University pharmacologist Raymond Woosley, who told *Science News*, "Can you believe it? . . . Why would you want to jump to another untested combination that might do the same thing?"

Quoted in Kathleen Fackelmann, "In the Wake of Fen-Phen," *Science News*, October 18, 1997, p. 253.

brought by victims of valvular heart disease and their families, who had banded together in a class-action lawsuit. As more people filed claims against the company (renamed Wyeth in 2002), the amount of money in the trust fund had to be increased several times in the years that followed.

By 2006, more than six hundred thousand plaintiffs had joined the class-action suit, and Wyeth's trust fund had reached $22 billion, although the company had paid out less than $2 billion. Approximately 50,000 fen-phen users, including those with PPH, have refused to settle through the class-action agreement and are pursuing individual lawsuits against the company.

After Fen-Phen

Although dieters can no longer take fen-phen, they can ask their doctors for prescriptions for several other kinds of diet drugs. The "phen" portion of fen-phen, or phentermine, remains on the market as a drug sold by generic pharmaceutical manufacturers. As a result, it carries a variety of brand names, including Ionamin, Adipex-P, and Fastin. The drug is supposed to be prescribed only for obese patients.

Another prescription drug being used to treat obesity is Prozac. Some doctors began to offer obese patients low doses of the medication after patients taking the drug to treat depression reported that it made them lose their appetite.

Similarly, after the antidepressant sibutramine was found to be an appetite suppressant, Abbott Laboratories began marketing it as a prescription diet drug called Meridia. The drug, which enhances both serotonin and norepinephrine, helps people eat less because it gives them the feeling of having eaten enough food. Tests have shown that it does not cause valvular disease or PPH, but it is not as effective in promoting weight loss as fen-phen. Most Meridia patients report losing no more than 10 pounds (4.5kg).

Even so, some people question the safety of Meridia. The consumer advocacy group Public Citizen has called for its

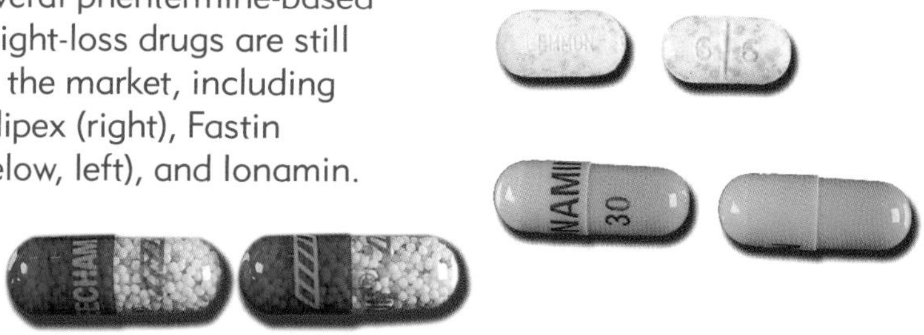

Several phentermine-based weight-loss drugs are still on the market, including Adipex (right), Fastin (below, left), and Ionamin.

withdrawal from the market, citing at least 29 deaths, mostly due to heart attacks, associated with the drug. However, because obesity also puts people at high risk for cardiac disease, and the Meridia warning label indicates that the drug can increase blood pressure, it remains on the market. Meridia is not approved for use by people with a history of high blood pressure or heart disease.

New Directions

Researchers took a new approach when they developed the prescription drug orlistat. Unlike fen-phen and sibutramine, which affect chemicals in the brain, orlistat works on food in the stomach. Marketed in the United States by GlaxoSmith Kline since 1999 under the brand name Xenical, orlistat was developed by Swiss drug maker Hoffman-La Roche. The drug causes weight loss because it prevents a stomach enzyme (called lipase) from breaking down the fat in foods. Instead of being digested and absorbed by the body, the undigested fat molecules pass through the intestines out of the body.

Clinical studies have shown that Xenical produces results nearly as good as those achieved with fen-phen. Researchers estimate that a dieter following a nutritious diet and exercise regimen who lost 10 pounds (4.5kg) without taking the medication would lose from 15 to 18 pounds (6.8kg to 8.1kg) if taking Xenical at the same time.

The medication has been shown to be a particularly effective diet drug for obese adolescents. In 2005, a study published by the *Journal of the American Medical Association* reported on Xenical use in a weight control program sponsored by the Weill Cornell Medical Center in New York City. Dr. Lou Aronne, director of the program, discussed the results on the CBS program *The Early Show*:

> In this study, the teens involved were heavier than 98 percent of the teenagers in the country . . . These were children who are at very high-risk for developing diabetes and other complications that we associate with obesity.
>
> The average teenager lost about 7 pounds compared to teenagers on a placebo. . . . The important point is that both groups were doing the diet and exercise program as well.[16]

Aronne added that he believed Xenical is "appropriate if . . . teenager[s] who [are] at risk for medical problems [are] making an effort to lose, they're doing everything they can, but they're not making progress. If that's the case, then medication may be of value."[17]

Unfortunately, Xenical can have adverse effects. Patients must eat a low-fat diet while taking the drug in order to avoid gastrointestinal problems such as diarrhea, gas, and,

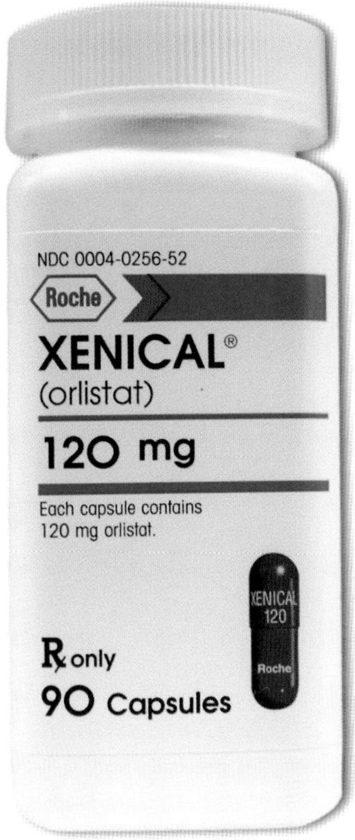

Available since 1999 as a prescription weight-loss aid, Xenical (orlistat) received preliminary approval from the FDA in 2006 to be sold at a reduced dosage as an over-the-counter drug.

sometimes, uncontrollable bowel movements. If a patient taking the drug consumes large amounts of fatty foods, the body cannot digest the fat, and severe diarrhea may result. Because Xenical also prevents the digestion of fat-soluble vitamins such as vitamins A, D, E, and K, doctors recommend that patients take vitamin supplements while they are on the drug.

In late 2005 GlaxoSmithKline applied to the FDA for approval of a low-dosage form of Xenical that would be sold without a prescription under the brand name Alli. The authorization to market this new over-the-counter diet drug received preliminary approval from the FDA in early 2006. If Alli receives approval for over-the-counter sales, GlaxoSmithKline plans to emphasize the need to include use of the drug as part of an overall weight-loss program. In fact, the name Alli was chosen because the drug is supposed to be *allied* with a weight-loss plan. In an interview with the *Los Angeles Times*, a vice president of GlaxoSmithKline Consumer Healthcare, Steven Burton, explained, "We want to develop [Alli] not just as a pill but as a program."[18]

Chapter 3

Weight-loss Dietary Supplements

In addition to prescription diet pills, weight-loss dietary supplements provide another option for dieters looking for help with their attempts to shed pounds. The weight-loss dietary supplement industry, which offers products that can be easily purchased over the counter and on the Internet, has grown quickly since the early 1990s. However, neither the safety of these products nor their effectiveness in promoting weight loss has been proven.

Dangers of PPA

Some over-the-counter weight-loss products may contain nonprescription drugs that have been approved by the Food and Drug Administration. Until 2000, two popular weight-loss products, Dexatrim and Acutrim, included an FDA-approved nonprescription drug called phenylpropanolamine, or PPA, as a major ingredient.

Like phentermine, PPA suppresses the appetite because it enhances the neurotransmitter norepinephrine in the brain. However, because the drug's effects on the neurotransmitter are mild, the Food and Drug Administration approved PPA's

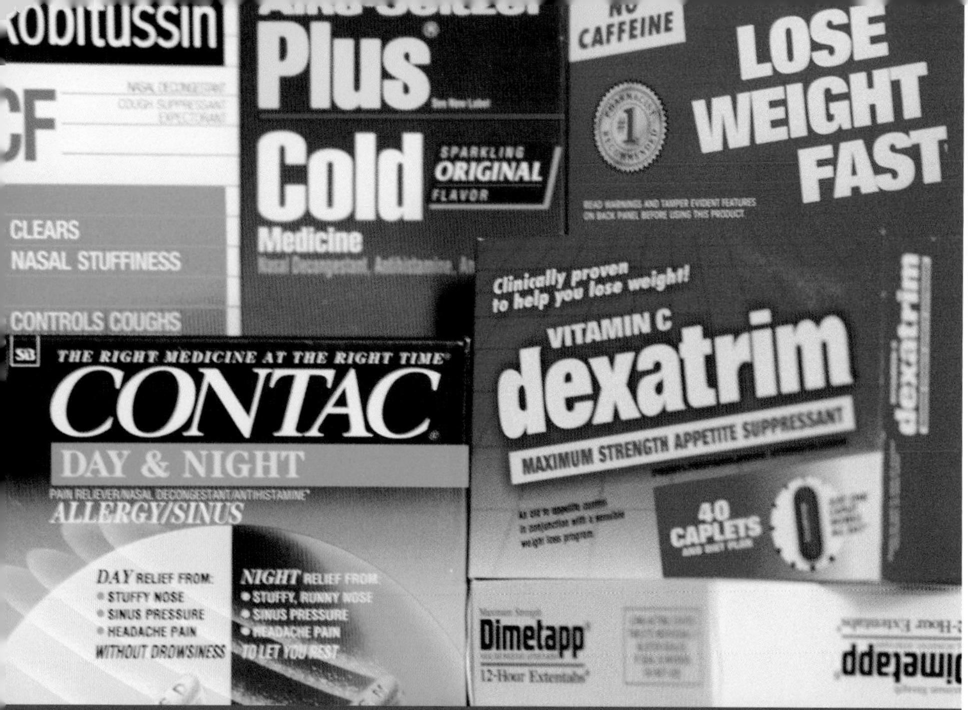

All of these nonprescription products used to contain phenylpropanolamine, or PPA. PPA was banned by the FDA in 2000 when studies showed it increased the risk of strokes.

use as a nonprescription drug. During the last quarter of the twentieth century, it was an ingredient in many over-the-counter products, including cold and flu remedies, as well as diet drugs.

However, in May 2000 the Food and Drug Administration learned of a study that showed PPA significantly increased the risk of hemorrhagic stroke (bleeding of the brain) in women. The following November, the FDA issued a public health advisory, asking manufacturers to remove phenylpropanolamine from their products.

Using Green Tea and Caffeine

With PPA no longer a viable ingredient, the manufacturers of weight-loss products such Dexatrim and Acutrim had to find a substitute. Many began using herbs and other dietary supplements in their formulations. For example, Dexatrim Results replaced PPA as its main ingredient with the herb ephedra. Then, when problems with ephedra arose, the manufacturer reformulated its diet drug once more, this time using green tea and caffeine.

Both green tea and caffeine are stimulants—meaning they speed up the body's metabolism and help people burn calories. The proponents of green tea claim it increases fat oxidation (that is, it helps burn fat). Caffeine, which is commonly found in tea, coffee, cocoa, and chocolate, is also a diuretic. It can reduce body weight because it decreases the amount of fluid in the body. Caffeine is frequently used in many over-the-counter weight-loss supplements. In fact, one of the ingredients in Acutrim is caffeine-rich chocolate.

Green tea and caffeine are among the main ingredients for the weight-loss aid Dexatrim Results. The manufacturer's Web site makes many claims about the various dietary supplements contained in the product:

> The formula is based on nutritional concepts that recognize your body's needs for vitamin and mineral replenishment as well as anti-oxidant support, especially when dieting and exercising. Like all Dexatrim dietary supplement formulas, it contains herbal extracts and minerals from around the world, which have been standardized and tested to insure quality.[19]

Other Dietary Supplements

Many of the "herbal extracts and minerals" found in Dexatrim are also used in other weight-loss products. Altogether, more than fifty different dietary supplements, derived from animals, plants, and minerals, serve as ingredients in more than 150 commercial weight-loss products being sold in the United States today.

One mineral commonly found in energy and diet drinks, powders, and pills is chromium. Manufacturers claim that chromium affects metabolism by helping the muscles use blood sugar more efficiently. The supplement is supposed to make people feel more energetic as it helps them metabolize foods more quickly. Because chromium's absorption in the body is enhanced when combined with picolinic acid, diet products often list this combined form (called chromium picolinate) as an ingredient.

The shells of crustaceans, such as shrimp and crabs, provide a dietary supplement called chitosan. The substance is supposed to prevent fat absorption in the intestines, so that undigested fat passes out of the body. Manufacturers using chitosan in weight-loss products often combine it with vitamin C and the digestive enzyme lipase, to enhance its effectiveness.

Herbal Products

Although minerals and animal-derived substances are used in some weight-loss aids, most products contain plant-based substances as main ingredients. Various plants and trees have had their components extracted, condensed into tablets, sealed in bottles, and sold under the claim that these substances can help people lose weight. Most are advertised as stimulants that increase metabolism and suppress the appetite.

One stimulant commonly found in weight-loss supplements is *citrus aurantium*, also known as bitter orange. Its active ingredient, synephrine, which is found in the dried outer peel of the fruit, is said to speed up the basal metabolic rate, boost energy, and help people burn calories faster. Bitter orange is combined with another stimulant, caffeine, in many weight-loss products.

Dietary supplements marketed as appetite suppressants have been harvested from areas around the world. Guggul, or guggulipid (which is extracted from the resin of the myrrh tree), comes from India. Brindleberry comes from the rind of the fruit of the Garcinia cambogia tree, which is found in Australia, Thailand, and southern India. St. John's wort is an herb that grows in the wild, and is commonly seen along highways and in meadows throughout North America.

Hoodia gordonii, which comes from a plant native to South Africa and Namibia, is also supposed to reduce the ap-

Taking Sweetness out of Sugar

A New Jersey company, Creator CCA Industries, is using the herb gymnema, found in the tropical forests of central and southern India, to take the taste out of sweet and sugary treats. The company uses the herb as the key ingredient of its SweetEnders tablets, lozenges, and gum.

The company suggests that people who want to kill their cravings for sugary treats take the SweetEnders supplement. According to the company, it will deaden a sweet tooth for up to two hours. "If you taste a chocolate bar, it's going to taste like cardboard," Creator CCA spokesperson Ana G. Lopo told *Newsday* in 2003. "It's kind of like a behavior modification approach."

Paul A. Lachance, a nutrition and food science professor at Rutgers University in New Jersey, told *Newsday* that the herb is probably safe for most consumers. However, the company stressed that SweetEnders is not a miracle diet drug. The product does nothing to kill the taste of fatty foods such as potato chips, cheeseburgers, or French fries.

Quoted in Dawn Wotapka, "SweetEnders: Herbal Help Curbing Sweet Cravings," *Newsday*, February 18, 2003, www.newday.com/nyp-dssupp3135248feb18,0,3593720.story

petite. It has been used for centuries by the indigenous people of the region—the Bushmen of the Kalahari Desert—because it helps them travel on long journeys with little food.

Not all plant and herbal dietary supplements used as weight-loss aids are stimulants. Many so-called dieters' teas contain substances that act as diuretics. These substances, which act as laxatives and cause fluid loss in the body, include senna, aloe, buckthorn, rhubarb root, and castor oil.

Celebrity Endorsement

Anybody can read about the benefits of green tea and other herbs by picking up the latest copies of celebrity or gossip magazines. They are often filled with stories of pop singers or movie stars claiming that certain products produce quick and easy ways to shed pounds. For example, model and reality TV star Anna Nicole Smith claimed that she lost 60 pounds (27.2kg) by taking the appetite suppressant TrimSpa. This weight-loss dietary supplement contains hoodia gordonii, green tea extract, and chromium, among other ingredients. "I decided to try taking TrimSpa because it said 'trim,'" Smith wrote in *Us* magazine in 2004. She explained:

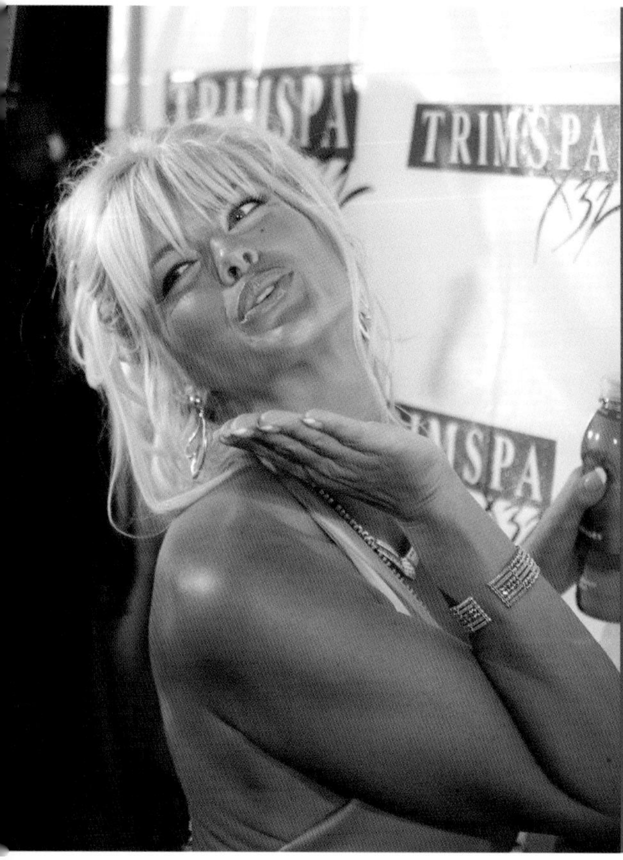

An enthusiastic spokesperson for the diet product TrimSpa, celebrity Anna Nicole Smith credits the product with helping her lose weight.

> I took six pills a day, which helped me eat a lot less. For breakfast, I would have either a handful of fruit, like melon, or oatmeal. The rest of the day I ate salad or more fruit. The first two weeks were really hard, but after that my usual cravings were gone. I used to order a pizza and eat half, or get eggs on a croissant with cheese and hash browns at Jack in the Box. Now that I actually enjoy eating healthier, the thought of [eating those junk foods] grosses me out!"[20]

Smith became such a fan of the product that she agreed to promote TrimSpa. Attaching a celebrity name to a product often can increase sales, and apparently Smith is an effective spokesperson. According to a November 2004 study of dietary supplements published in *American Family Physician*, TrimSpa and its competitors sell some $1.3 billion worth of weight-loss supplements a year to American consumers.

Some Scientific Support to the Claims

Sales of weight-loss aids increase when people believe the products they are buying actually work. However, there have not been many scientific studies on the effectiveness of dietary supplements, although a few researchers have reported results that appear to support weight-loss claims. For example, a 1999 Swiss study showed that six out of ten men who took capsules containing extract of green tea burned eighty more calories a day than they did when not taking the substance.

An older study, published in 1981 by University of Southern Colorado psychology professor Paul J. Kulkosky, has been cited to support the theory that caffeine acts as an appetite suppressant. Kulkosky documented the results of feeding caffeine to lab rats and concluded, "a prominent finding in the present study is that orally consumed caffeine strongly suppresses feeding behavior."[21]

In their book, *The Caffeine Advantage*, authors Bennett Alan Weinberg and Bonnie K. Bealer noted the weight-loss capabilities of caffeine. They wrote, "It delays the onset of hunger, and taking it before meals reduces the amount of food you need to feel full."[22]

Concerns About Effectiveness

However, despite the pronouncements of celebrities and claims from certain scientists about the effectiveness of weight-loss dietary supplement aids, most medical researchers believe that the products do not work. In response to the Swiss study on the weight-loss benefits of green tea, Professor Jeffrey Blumberg of Tufts University, in Massachusetts, explained that the study's findings did not prove that green tea would actually help people lose weight. In the Tufts University *Health and Nutrition Letter*, Blumberg stated that an obese person who needs to shed 100 pounds (45.3kg) or more would not benefit from burning an extra eighty calories a day. That kind of weight loss would be so minimal, he said, it "could easily be undone by eating a single cookie or a handful of chips."[23]

The manufacturers of weight-loss products made with dietary supplements may claim their products provide results. However, they seldom can point to scientifically accepted research that supports those assertions.

Concerns About Safety

Because dietary supplements are substances that can be found in nature, they are often advertised as "natural," a label that consumers often assume means "safe." But natural substances can be dangerous when they are contaminated, consumed in large amounts, or used over long periods of time.

Some researchers have found weight-loss dietary substances contaminated with heavy metals, pesticides, or other toxic ingredients. Some weight-loss aids containing guggulipid have been tainted by lead. One chromium-based dietary supplement was reported to contain traces of hexavalent chromium, a toxic form of the mineral, instead of the commonly used supplement, chromium picolinate.

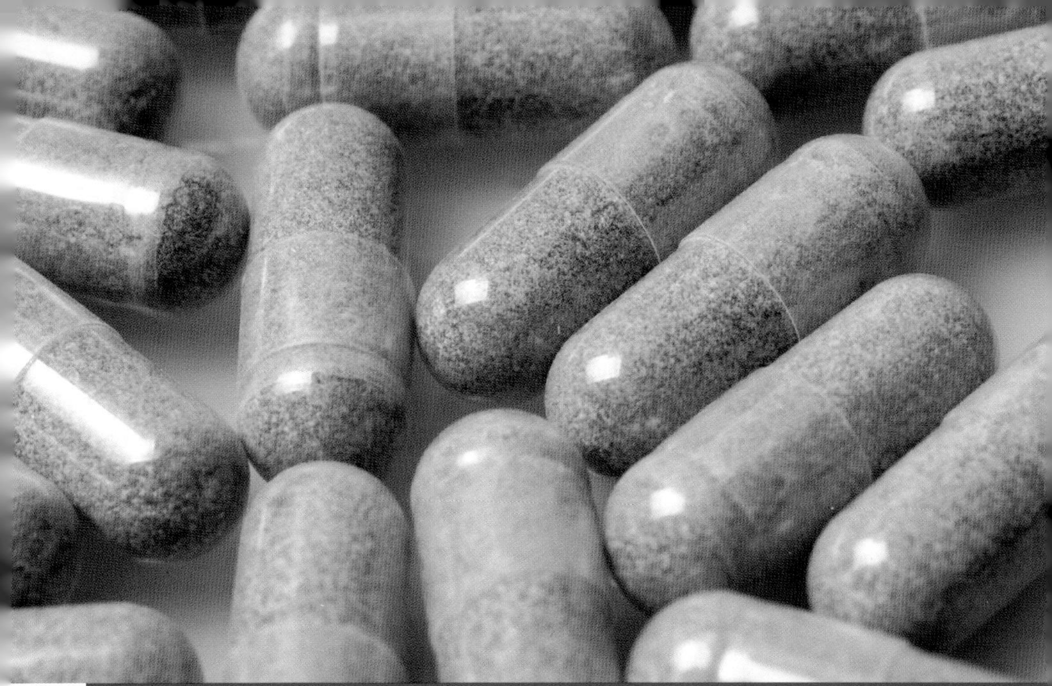

One concern about dietary supplements is that manufacturers do not have to meet FDA standards regarding the strength of ingredients or the purity of their products.

Some products may provide much greater amounts of ingredients than the label indicates. Large amounts of certain dietary supplements could exacerbate existing medical problems or cause new health problems. For example, in large doses, chromium can cause anemia, liver dysfunction, kidney failure, memory loss, and even cancer. When taken in high doses, brindleberry has been found to cause breast milk to dry up in pregnant women.

Long-term consumption of certain products can also be dangerous, particularly if they contain large amounts of a dietary supplement. For example, some weight-loss supplements and energy drinks can contain extremely high amounts of caffeine—as much as five times more than the amount found in a cup of black coffee (typically about 135 milligrams). Such high dosages of caffeine have been shown to cause complications such as heart palpitations, headaches, insomnia, and anxiety.

In an interview broadcast on CNN *Daybreak*, nutritionist Lisa Drayer commented that a single dose of the weight-loss

Operation Waistline

Many weight-loss dietary supplements are advertised with unproven claims like "Lose weight without exercise!" or "Never diet again!" Monitoring for truth in advertising falls under the control of a government agency called the U.S. Federal Trade Commission (FTC). It can force manufacturers to stop advertising their products as something they are not. Since 1997, the FTC has run Operation Waistline, which polices advertising of weight-loss products. In spite of the agency's efforts, the FTC reports that 40 percent of ads for weight-loss products published in newspapers and magazines in 2002 made at least one false representation.

Through Operation Waistline, the FTC has fined numerous manufacturers and forced the withdrawal of product ads that make false claims. Still, with hundreds of weight-loss products on the market, FTC officials admit that the agency lacks the resources to ensure that all advertising about weight-loss products is truthful.

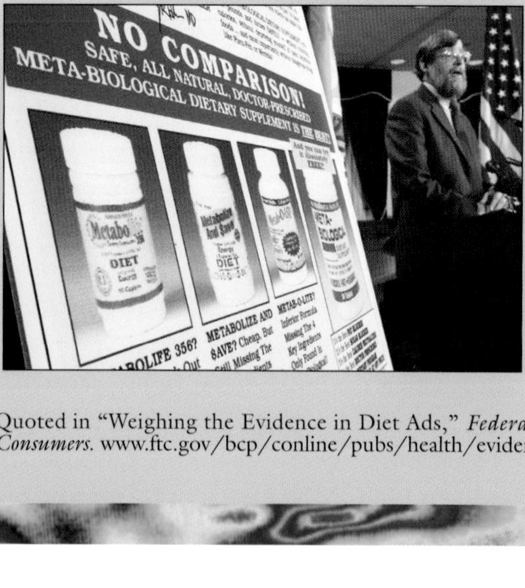

Howard Beales, director of the FTC's Bureau of Consumer Protection, announces in July 2003 that three manufacturers of weight-loss products will face penalties for making false advertising claims.

Quoted in "Weighing the Evidence in Diet Ads," *Federal Trade Commission: Facts for Consumers*. www.ftc.gov/bcp/conline/pubs/health/evidence.htm.

product Dexatrim contains about two-thirds the amount of the caffeine found in a cup of coffee. Users are instructed to take three tablets per day, which amounts to 240 milligrams daily. Drayer expressed concern as to whether that much caffeine is healthy: "Each tablet contains 80 milligrams of caffeine. You take three per day, you're going to feel a jolt. And . . . the label warns not to take it if you start to experience headaches, dizziness or shortness of breath."[24]

Caffeine is also mildly addictive. Without regular doses of caffeine in the morning and throughout the day, coffee drinkers may feel drowsy, irritable, and unable to concentrate. And, caffeine's addictive qualities become apparent if a person stops using caffeine altogether. Coffee drinkers can experience withdrawal symptoms, such as long-lasting and severe headaches that continue for as long as a week.

Long-term use of green tea—which contains a small amount of caffeine—has also been accompanied by adverse effects. Regular use can cause insomnia, nervousness, hyperactivity, increased blood pressure, headaches, vertigo, increased heart rate, and heartburn.

Even short-term use of some weight-loss dietary supplements has been linked to health risks. Bitter orange has been reported by some users to cause hypertension (high blood pressure) or arrhythmias (disturbances in heart rhythm) that can lead to heart attack, stroke, and even death. Guggul has been shown to cause diarrhea, nausea, and skin rashes. People who take St. John's wort may suffer numerous adverse effects, including nausea, constipation, skin rashes and hives, insomnia, dizziness, confusion, and irregular breathing. The herb has also been shown to interact with other medications, and can be poisonous if taken with certain prescription drugs.

Insufficient Research

With newly discovered substances, very little is known about potential adverse effects. In 2003, after being featured on several news stories, hoodia gordonii was rushed into the marketplace as an ingredient in various weight-loss products. No studies supported the effectiveness of the substance at the time. Even two years later, when the *New York Times* asked nutrition specialist Dr. Jonathan Waitman whether he thought people should take hoodia gordonii, he replied, "In good conscience, I can't recommend something when the benefits are unproven and the health risks are unknown."[25]

In this case, few studies of hoodia gordonii existed because its use as an ingredient in a weight-loss supplement was so new. However, because rigorous testing of dietary supplements is not required by law, most dietary supplements have undergone little scientific study.

Ongoing Controversy

Most people do not stop to think about whether the diet supplement they are taking is safe or effective. They just want help losing weight. In an article on common weight-loss supplements published in the November 2004 issue of *American Family Physician*, Drs. Robert Saper, David Eisenberg, and Russell Phillips explained:

> These supplements appeal to the desire for a "magic bullet" that is less demanding than special diets and increased physical activity. They are available without a prescription and often advertise remarkable benefits. Patients may also be attracted to them because they are marketed as "natural," which may be interpreted by some (albeit inaccurately) as an assurance of safety and efficacy.[26]

The authors conclude their review by saying that physicians should recommend only those products that have met sound criteria:

> If there is strong evidence for a product's quality, safety, and efficacy, it may be reasonable to *recommend* that product and closely monitor the patient. No supplements discussed in this review meet these criteria, how-

ever. In contrast, it would be appropriate to *discourage* use of products when there is strong evidence for lack of quality, safety, or efficacy.[27]

In response, proponents of weight-loss supplements argue that the products cause few severe adverse effects. They note that some common herbal supplements have served as dietary aids in certain cultures for hundreds, and even thousands of years. If hoodia gordonii is dangerous, they ask, how could the people of the Kalahari Desert have survived on the herb for so long?

The American Herbal Products Association, which represents the manufacturers of many weight-loss supplements, reinforced this position by making the following statement: "The safety of herbal products as a general class has been well established by both their long history of traditional use

Although some dietary supplements may carry warning labels, such as the one below, manufacturers of these products are not yet required by law to include such disclaimers.

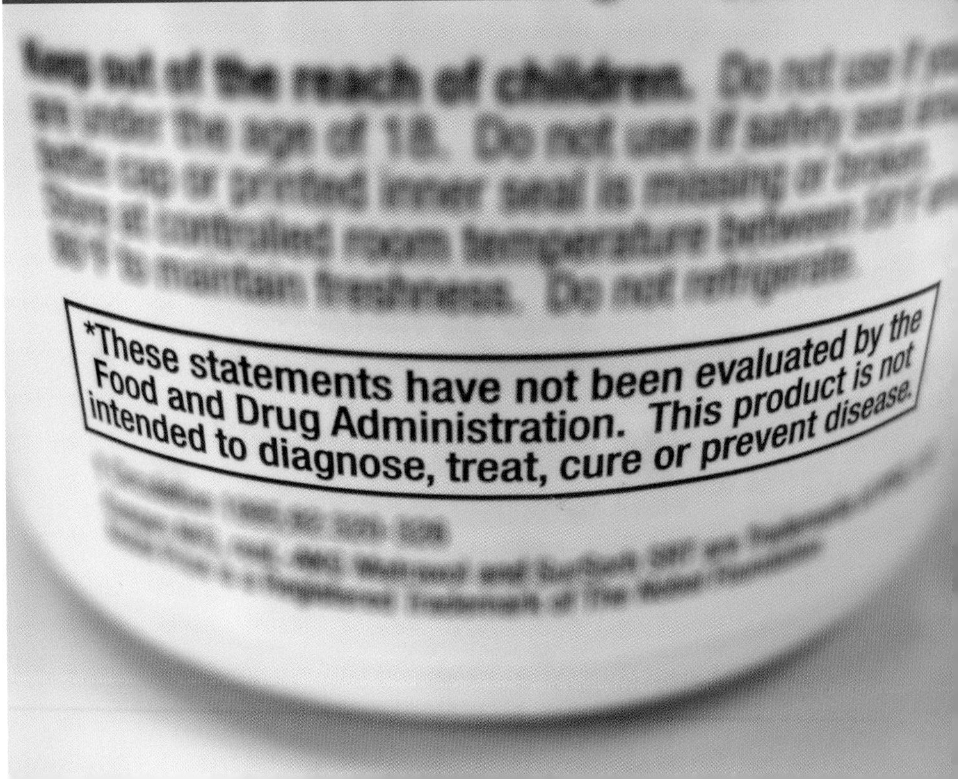

worldwide and by their broad contemporary use by a significant proportion of the population, estimated to be nearly half of the U.S. population."[28]

Government Regulation

Just because millions of people take dietary supplements does not mean they are safe. Many physicians hesitate to recommend their use because of the continuing lack of scientific proof that these substances work. But these studies are not being done because of the 1994 Dietary Supplement Health and Education Act (DSHEA).

DSHEA established a legal definition of dietary supplements as natural substances. The law called for FDA approval of a dietary supplement or product only if its label claims that it prevents, treats, or cures a specific disease or health condition. Because of DSHEA, the FDA does not have the legal authority to monitor the manufacture of dietary supplements or to establish quality control (to ensure ingredient strength, uniformity, and purity) in any product that contains them.

If a problem with a dietary supplement occurs, the FDA has the authority to remove it from the market. However, to do so, the federal agency (and not the manufacturer) must prove the supplement is dangerous.

Playing Russian Roulette

Some scientists and consumer advocates believe that the federal government needs to take a stronger role in the regulation of dietary supplements. During an interview broadcast in 2000 on National Public Radio's *Talk of the Nation*, Bruce Silverglade, the director of legal affairs for the public interest group Center for Science in the Public Interest, described the consequences of the Dietary Supplement Health and Education Act:

> Before 1994, the FDA had the authority to require that dietary supplement ingredients be demonstrated to be

"Before" and "After" Pictures

Those "before" and "after" pictures that dietary supplements manufacturers feature in their advertisements are often fraudulent, according to the U.S. Federal Trade Commission (FTC). A 2002 FTC report entitled *Weight Loss Advertising: An Analysis of Current Trends* indicated that 42 percent of published advertisements and TV commercials for weight-loss supplements featured such photos. The agency raised doubts as to the authenticity of many of them.

In its review of the ads, the FTC found that the typical "before" picture often features a "snapshot quality photograph of the subject that incorporates poor posture, neutral facial expression, unkempt hair, unfashionable attire, poor lighting, and washed out skin tones." The "after" picture is a "brightly lit (sometimes studio portrait quality) pose of smiling subject in fashionable, often skimpy, attire, shoulders held back, tummy tucked in, with a stylish hair style and carefully applied makeup."

The FTC reports that the same person usually does not appear in both photos. The head of the obese subject in the "before" picture is often digitally replaced with the head of the slender subject in the "after" pose.

Quoted in Richard L. Cleland, et al., *Weight-Loss Advertising: An Analysis of Current Trends*. Washington: U.S. Federal Trade Commission, 2002, p. 12.

safe before they were sold. Because of industry lobbying, the FDA lost that authority, Congress deregulated the industry, and now dietary supplement ingredients can be sold before they are demonstrated to be safe. So essentially, consumers are playing Russian roulette. I think one thing that we can agree on is that many

> dietary supplements can be beneficial and have health benefits, but like drugs, they can also carry health risks . . . as it stands now, the FDA's hands are tied.[29]

There is some movement in Congress to provide the FDA with more authority in regulating dietary supplements. In 2003, Senator Richard Durbin of Illinois introduced the Dietary Supplements Safety Act—legislation that requires, among other conditions, that dietary supplement manufacturers report serious adverse events to the FDA. That same year U.S. Representative Susan Davis of California introduced the Dietary and Supplement Access and Awareness Act, which requires manufacturers to submit a list of their weight-loss supplements and ingredients to the FDA every six months.

In the law proposed by Davis, the FDA would gain the power to require dietary supplement manufacturers to demonstrate that their products are safe. The law would provide the agency with the authority to inspect the manufacturers' records to ensure they are not concealing evidence that their products caused harm. Armed with that information, Davis said, the FDA would have the tools to order an unsafe weight-loss supplement pulled from the market. In a statement issued on the floor of the U.S. House, Davis described the benefits of this law:

> With this information in hand, the FDA can make sensible, informed decisions and policies about dietary supplements. Consumers can have greater assurance than they currently do about the safety of the products on the market. We cannot continue to stand on the sidelines and let this serious public health threat go unchecked.[30]

The makers of dietary supplements and products containing these substances disagree about the need for any legislation. Efforts to prevent passage have effectively prevented these bills from being brought to a vote.

Chapter 4

Ephedra and Its Dangers

One of the most controversial dietary supplements is ephedra, also known by its Chinese name, ma huang. Despite being linked to health problems and many deaths, the substance remained on the market in the United States for many years because the Food and Drug Administration could not definitively prove that it is dangerous. Fans of the dietary supplement continue to insist ephedra is effective and safe when used correctly, while family members of its victims continue to call for a complete ban of the substance.

A Replacement for Amphetamine

Used for centuries in China as a traditional herbal medicine, ephedra contains ephedrine, which scientists combined with other chemicals to synthesize the drug amphetamine. After physicians stopped writing prescriptions for amphetamine-based diet pills in the 1970s, athletes began using ephedra-based bodybuilding aids and energy boosters because they produced a similar effect. The herbal supplements were marketed in gyms and health food stores, as well as in advertisements in weight-lifting magazines. Athletes found the

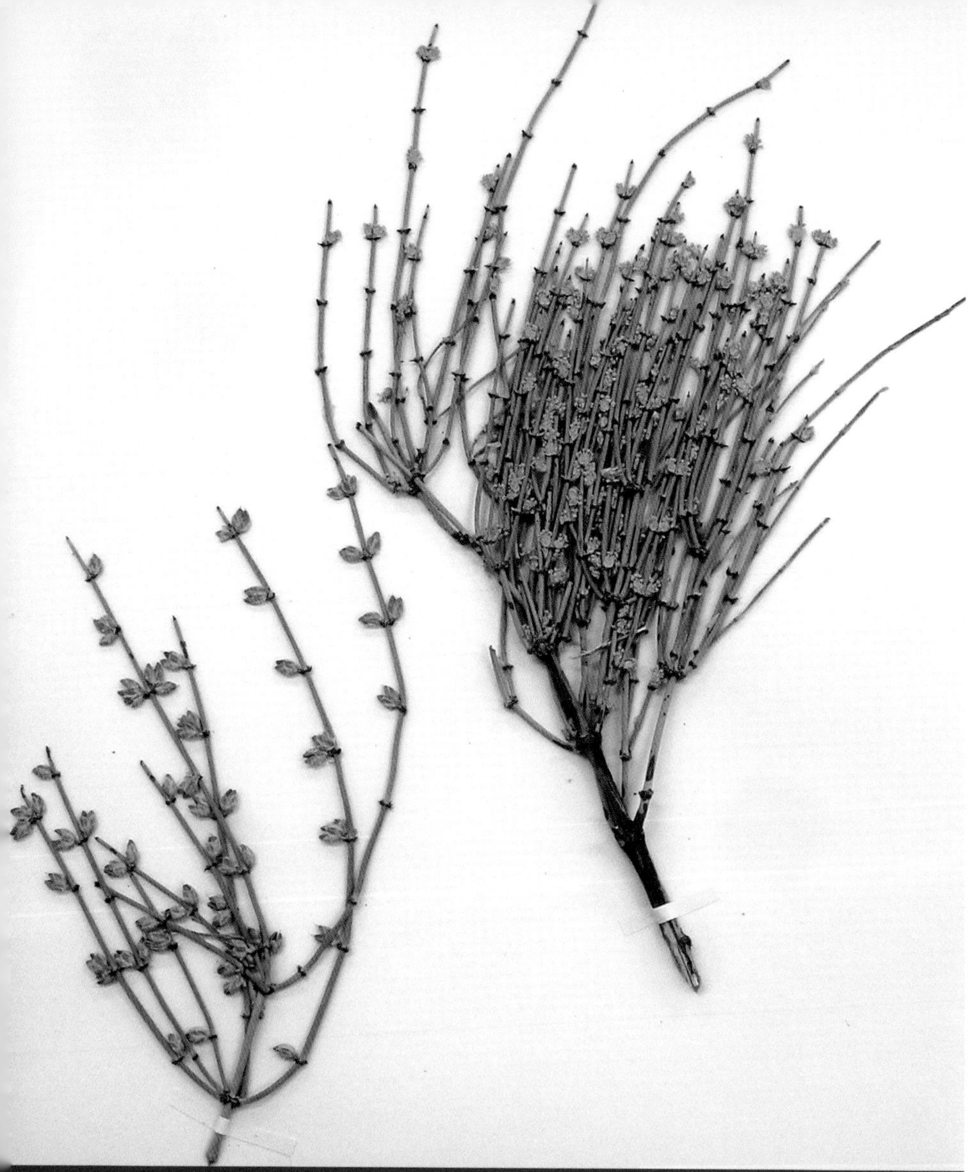

The herb ephedra is a stimulant that reduces appetite. However, its use in dietary supplements has been linked to numerous deaths.

ephedrine stimulants helped them increase their endurance, as well as burn calories.

During the early 1990s, the herb also started showing up as the active ingredient in "all-natural," over-the-counter weight-loss supplements. Millions of people purchased ephedra-based products such as Metabolife 356, Ripped Fuel, and Up Your Gas because they believed the products were energy boosters that would also help them lose fat and build muscle. Few realized they were consuming a substance that could be fatal.

Early Warnings

As growing numbers of people took ephedra-based diet drugs and other products, the Food and Drug Administration began to receive reports of adverse effects linked to the use of herbal supplements. By the mid-1990s approximately four hundred adverse reactions had been reported, including fifteen fatalities.

One of those who died after taking ephedra was George Korizis, a graduate student at Tufts University in Massachusetts. An avid exerciser who did not smoke or drink, Korizis had been taking Ripped Fuel before workouts to boost his energy and stamina. An autopsy found that Korizis' heart was riddled with bits of dead tissue, a result commonly seen with the use of stimulants.

By 1996 the FDA had received numerous reports that linked health problems and deaths with ephedra use. But under the restrictions imposed in 1994 by the U.S. Dietary Supplement Health and Education Act, the FDA could not immediately call for a ban of ephedra. Instead, the agency had to build a case against the herb, proving that it caused harm. In the case of ephedra, the effort would take years.

No Quality Control

As researchers turned their attention to ephedra, the inability of the FDA to ensure the quality and content of dietary supplements became apparent. In 2000, chemist Bill Gurley, a researcher with the University of Arkansas for Medical Sciences tested various dietary supplements to determine whether the amount of ephedra listed on the labels matched their actual content. Gurley discovered there was a wide variance between what the labels said was in the tablets and what was truly contained in each dose. He found that the tablets of one ephedra-based weight-loss supplement, called Exandra Lean, actually contained no ephedra at all.

When Gurley questioned the Exandra Lean manufacturer about the missing ingredient, he was told that the company's supplier had produced the pills without ephedra. Although aware that its product did not contain the labeled ingredient, the manufacturer continued to sell Exandra Lean anyway.

Just as it is possible for one bottle of a dietary supplement to contain no ephedra, there is also the chance that another bottle could contain much more ephedra than the label indicates. This lack of quality control increases the potential for a consumer to overdose on a supplement and suffer a serious, and possibly fatal, adverse reaction.

George Washington University health policy analyst Thomas J. Moore notes that safety concerns should dictate better quality control over dietary supplement products: "Dietary supplements don't meet the level of standards that my hair dryer has to meet," he complains. "Everywhere [else] you go, everything you touch, from pumping gas to turning on your hair dryer, there is a web of consumer safety."[31]

Inconsistent Dosing

Many physicians are concerned that patient-self dosing of dietary supplements containing stimulants like ephedra holds danger as well. People taking dietary aids are essentially self-medicating themselves—taking whatever doses they desire without first consulting their doctors or even paying much attention to what the labels suggest.

However, with ephedra, FDA researchers learned, adverse effects occurred regardless of the amount being taken. In an interview with National Public Radio, former FDA Commissioner Jane Henney explained,

> What we saw in the data was that people were taking different doses of the product. It didn't seem to matter

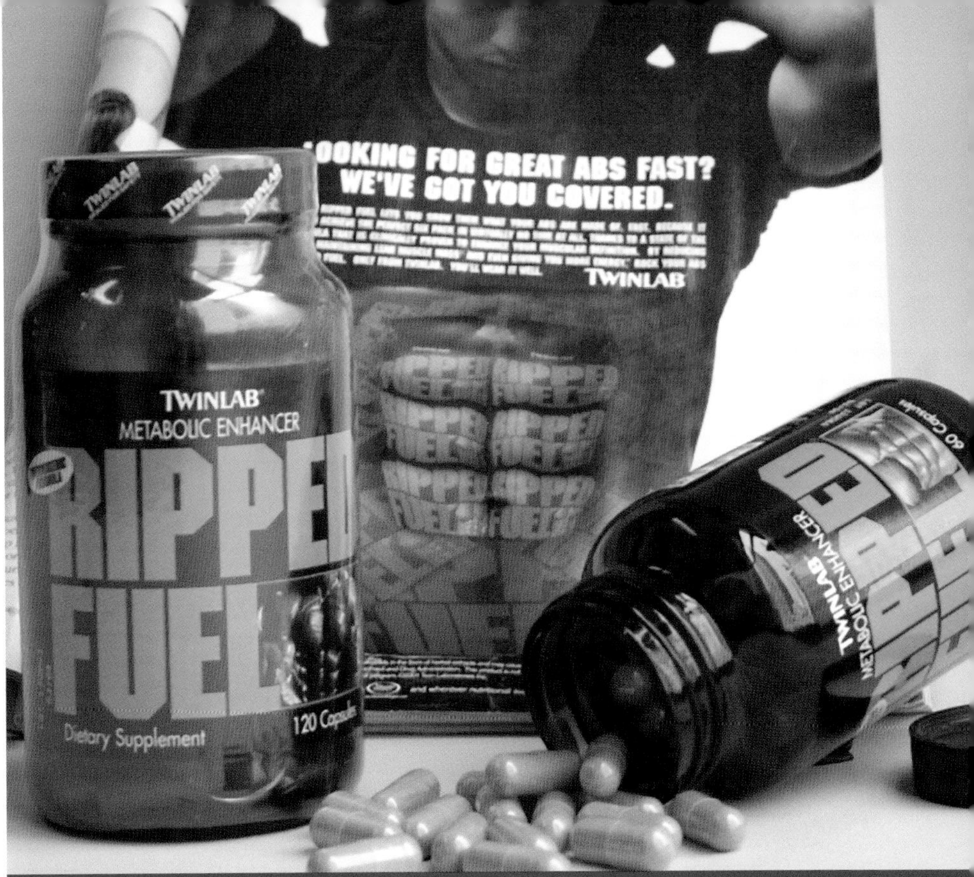

The safety of ephedra-based products such as Ripped Fuel, which has been linked to the deaths of several athletes, continues to be debated.

whether you were on a very low dose or high dose, whether you were young and healthy. Almost without warning this product could be a cause for concern, and the risks could be severe, anywhere from heart attacks to strokes to death.[32]

A Deadly Result

Despite mounting evidence that ephedra posed serious health risks, the dietary supplements industry stepped up its production of over-the-counter weight-loss aids that included the herb. Many manufacturers began using ephedra in their formulations to replace PPA after it was banned in 2000. But soon two well-publicized incidents made the public begin to question the safety of ephedra.

In 2001, while working out on the practice field, Minnesota Vikings lineman Korey Stringer suddenly collapsed and died from heatstroke. Heatstroke occurs when body temperature drastically soars above normal (98.6° Fahrenheit, or 37° Celsius) to temperatures as high as 110°F (43°C). Symptoms of heatstroke come on quickly: the skin loses moisture, and the dizzy, nauseous victim has trouble breathing. In some cases, as in Stringer's, heatstroke can be fatal. It was determined that the football player had been using Ripped Fuel, the same ephedra-based weight-loss supplement consumed by Korizis.

Another professional athlete was similarly struck down two years later. During spring training, while working out in the

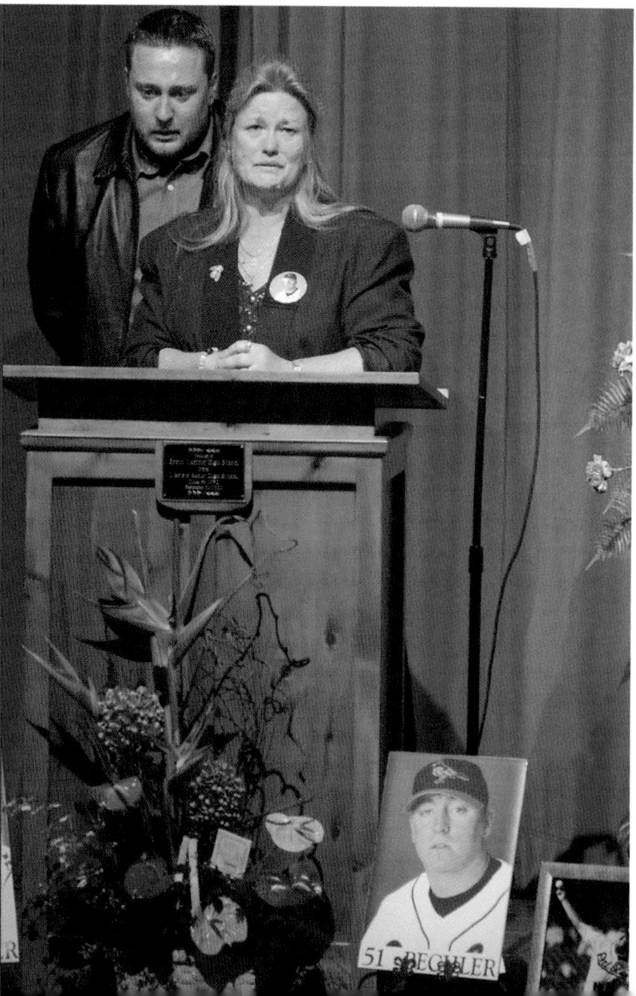

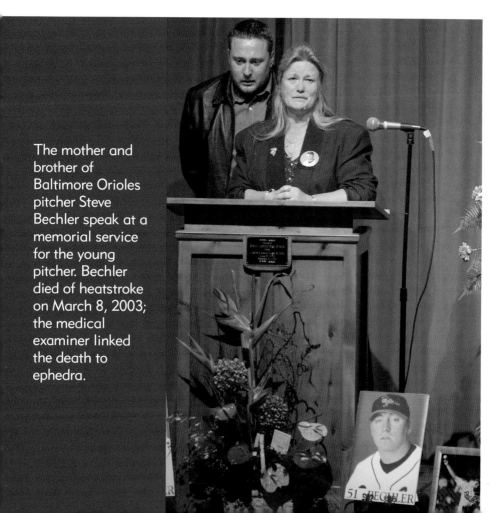

The mother and brother of Baltimore Orioles pitcher Steve Bechler speak at a memorial service for the young pitcher. Bechler died of heatstroke on March 8, 2003; the medical examiner linked the death to ephedra.

hot Florida sun, Baltimore Orioles pitcher Steve Bechler died of heatstroke. He had been taking Xenadrine RFA-1, an over-the-counter weight-loss supplement that contained ephedra. Bechler suffered from no other ailment that would have contributed to his death, Bechler family attorney David Meiselman told CNN. "Steve was a healthy young man," Meiselman insisted:

> He was healthy enough to pitch Major League Baseball. He had passed a rigorous physical examination, conducted by a medical doctor for the Baltimore Orioles, and it would seem to me that a 23-year-old Major League Baseball pitcher, who is healthy enough to play for the Baltimore Orioles, should be healthy enough to take an over-the-counter weight loss pill. . . . I believe that when it all is said and done, it will be proven, overwhelmingly, that ephedra was the cause of Steve's death.[33]

Widespread Use Among Athletes

Ephedra has been shown to interfere with the body's ability to regulate heat, which can cause elevated body temperature—the condition that led to the deaths of Stringer and Bechler. Because ephedra is a stimulant, it can also cause high blood pressure, heart palpitations, and heart attacks. Its use has been linked to strokes and seizures, even in apparently healthy young adults.

Many dietary supplements include a mix of ephedra and caffeine. Together, the two substances have proven to be a particularly potent calorie burner. However, the stimulating qualities of the ephedra-caffeine combination can also be deadly, particularly when taken by people with a history of high blood pressure or heart problems. The dietary supplement products that Stringer and Bechler took before they died were actually ephedra-caffeine cocktails.

High school athletes have also turned to ephedra and caffeine to give them a competitive edge. A member of the wrestling and football teams for his Lincoln, Illinois, high school in 2002, Sean Riggins would prepare for each competition by swallowing a dietary supplement known as Yellow Jacket, which contained twenty-five milligrams of ephedra and three hundred milligrams of caffeine. He usually drank a high-caffeine beverage, such as Mountain Dew or Red Bull, along with the pill.

In September 2002, shortly before a football game, Sean consumed the ephedra and caffeine combination in what he called the "jacketing" ritual. That night, he was too ill to play in the game. The next day, he saw a doctor, who diagnosed Sean's illness as a case of the flu. Later that day, Sean suffered a heart attack and died. Chuck Fricke, the coroner who performed the autopsy on Sean's body, told *Sports Illustrated*, "Basically his heart was pumping so fast, it gave out on him."[34]

Despite the negative publicity, many people continued to use ephedra-based products. The football strength and conditioning coach at Southern Methodist University in Texas, Chuck Faucette, told *Sports Illustrated* in 2003, "Everyone, and I mean everyone, takes supplements now. When a recruit comes in, the first question I get is, 'What kind of supplements can I take?'"[35]

Attempts to Ban Ephedra

As reports of deaths linked to ephedra spread, some professional sports leagues reacted by banning their players from using the substance. In 2002 the National Football League stated that players using ephedra would be suspended for four games—the same penalty they would suffer for consuming anabolic steroids and similar performance-enhancing drugs. Other athletic organizations, including the National Collegiate Athletic Association (NCAA) and the International Olympic Committee have also prohibited players from using ephedra. In announcing its ban, the International Olympic Committee cited evidence suggesting ephedra is addictive, although scientific studies have not supported that claim.

Ephedra's Psychiatric Effect

In addition to ephedra's adverse physiological effects, psychological problems have also been attributed to use of the drug. In January 2005 researchers reported in the *American Journal of Psychiatry* that of 1,820 reports of adverse reactions linked to ephedra, 57 cases also included episodes of mental illness. Mental disorders that occurred in patients taking ephedra included psychosis, a severe disorder in which an individual exhibits irrational behavior, as well as depression, hallucinations, sleep disturbance, and suicidal thoughts. The study's researchers determined that in most cases where the users already had some degree of mental illness, the ephedra enhanced their symptoms.

During a 2002 U.S. Senate hearing on ephedra use, California resident Karen Ruiz testified that she started taking ephedra to lose weight. However, within a week she had to be hospitalized in a psychiatric institution. She recalled, "I remember I was suddenly feeling very aware of a spiritual realm. And at one point, I felt that I was being watched. And I remember thinking my neighbor was demonically possessed. I was flipping in and out of paranoia."

U.S. Senate Committee on Governmental Affairs, *Hearings on When Diets Turn Deadly: Consumer Safety and Weight Loss Supplements*, July 31, 2002.

Some NFL players protested the football league's official ban. Unconvinced that ephedra is dangerous, they insisted they would continue taking it. In November 2002 Carolina Panthers defensive lineman Julius Peppers received a four-game suspension after testing positive for ephedra. In 2003 Byron Chamberlain of the Minnesota Vikings and Lee

The use of dietary supplements to improve performance on the playing field has been reported among athletes of all ages, including football players in middle school and high school.

Flowers of the Denver Broncos were suspended for similar offenses. That year, running back Marshall Faulk of the St. Louis Rams told *Sports Illustrated* that ephedra was so important to his training regimen that he intended to keep taking it despite the ban. John Welbourn of the Philadelphia Eagles also complained, saying, "The NFL basically scapegoated ephedra. The Chinese have been taking it for two thousand years. It's stupid."[36]

Major League Baseball did not ban ephedra use despite the well-publicized deaths. Some baseball players insisted that when taken in modest doses, ephedra could be an effective

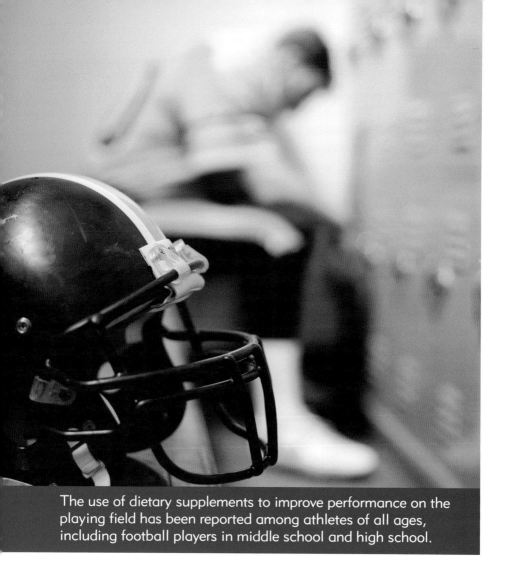

weight-loss supplement. Bechler's teammate, Orioles outfielder Jay Gibbons, told an interviewer for *PR Newswire* that he had used an ephedra-based supplement to help him lose 15 pounds (6.8kg) prior to spring training in 2002. He said, "It's a good supplement if taken right. I've never had any problems with it. I've never had any dizziness with it. It's just like caffeine."[37]

Other baseball players took the tragedies of Stringer and Bechler more seriously. Before Bechler's death, New York Mets catcher Mike Piazza had praised an ephedra-based supplement, telling an interviewer that "Ripped Fuel is kind of cool." Following the Baltimore Oriole pitcher's death, though, Piazza said he stopped using the supplement. "I just used it a couple of times," said Piazza. "And this was before the guy [died]. Obviously, I wouldn't recommend it now."[38]

In Defense of Ephedra

During the early 2000s, the FDA continued to build a case for a comprehensive national ban on ephedra. The federal agency encountered strong opposition from the supplements industry, which insisted that when used properly ephedra was safe and effective. The industry cited a 2002 study by the New York Obesity Research Center of St. Luke's-Roosevelt Hospital that had reported ephedra, in limited dosages, helped patients lose weight. The eighty-three obese patients who participated in the study over a six-month period each lost an average of about 12 pounds (5.4kg). In contrast, patients who followed the same regimen without taking ephedra each lost an average of only about 6 pounds (2.7kg).

The St. Luke's-Roosevelt study also suggested that the herbal supplement's side effects were not as serious as some believed. Many of the obese patients taking ephedra reported mild symptoms of heartburn, dry mouth, and insomnia, as well as modest increases in pulse rate. In addition, the physicians monitoring the study participants found no evidence that consuming the herb weakened patients' hearts.

Advocates for the dietary supplements industry argued that most people who experienced serious adverse reactions after taking ephedra had misused the herb or had weak hearts to begin with. Steven Karch, a California physician who serves as a consultant to the Ephedra Education Council (which is supported by the dietary supplements industry) told *U.S. News and World Report*, "The only cases I know where people [who took ephedra] died, they had severe coronary artery disease or they took overdoses."[39]

The FDA Builds Its Case

Despite evidence from the St. Luke's-Roosevelt study, government regulators remained concerned about ephedra and its dangers. In building its case against the substance, the FDA asked five independent physicians to evaluate reports of adverse events it had received from consumers of dietary supplements. One evaluator, Dr. Raymond Woosley of Georgetown University in Washington, D.C., reported that 104 of the 140 cases reported to the FDA from 1977 to 1999 directly resulted from the patients' use of ephedra. Adverse reactions included strokes, heart attacks, seizures, and episodes of hypertension. Medical authorities elsewhere were also studying ephedra. In 2002 Canadian health authorities recommended that its citizens avoid consuming ephedra-based weight-loss supplements.

Some dietary supplement manufacturers responded to the alarms raised by medical experts and government officials by dropping ephedra as an ingredient in their formulations. They replaced it with other herbs and substances, including green tea, caffeine, and hoodia gordonii.

Before recommending a total ban on ephedra in the United States, the FDA proposed that dietary supplement manufacturers limit the amount of ephedra in each dose to 8 milligrams, taken no more than three times per day (or a daily dose of 24 mg). The federal agency also asked manufacturers to include labeling that indicated possible adverse effects and that instructed consumers not to take ephedra for longer than a week. However, the manufacturers opposed these restrictions. They had been telling ephedra users to take the dietary supplements for a period of three months. Clearly, adherence to the FDA's rules would have drastically reduced sales.

In 2002, 2003, and 2004 the U.S. House and Senate held a series of hearings on the safety of dietary supplements. During the hearings, several witnesses, including college student Greg Davis, testified about how ephedra had affected their lives. Davis testified that he started using an ephedra supplement while in high school. He hoped it would help him improve his performance on the football team so he could win a college scholarship and eventually turn pro. But at age sixteen Davis, testified, he started suffering seizures. One occurred while he was driving, he explained: "I got in a pretty

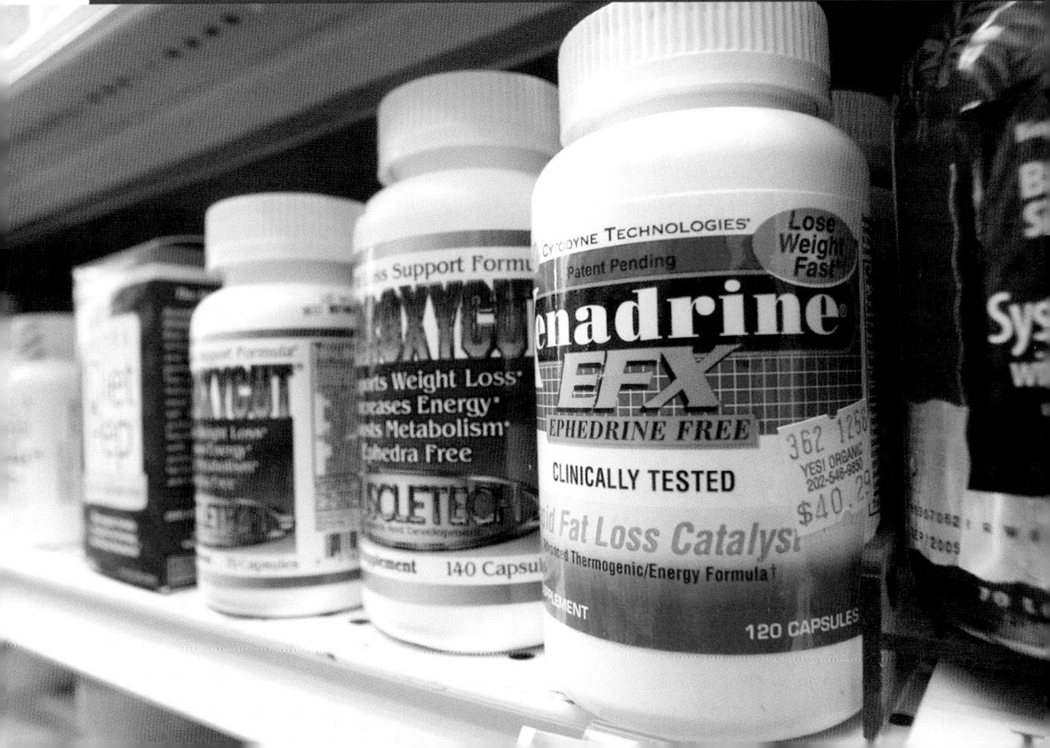

Fearing an FDA ban, some supplement manufacturers began to offer ephedrine-free dietary aids, such as the products pictured here. However, there is little evidence that these alternatives have any effect on weight loss.

bad car accident. My car veered off the right side of the road, ran through a guardrail and came to rest against a tree."[40]

In the hospital, a blood test indicated that Davis was under the influence of amphetamines, which was not the case. He explained that it was the ephedra in his system that registered as the illegal substance:

> When [hospital workers] did the blood test, my blood came up positive for amphetamines. You know, it's in the street drug, speed. At that time, I started to put two and two together and realized that the Ephedra, the so-called safe performance-enhancing supplement that I easily got off the Internet caused me to have these seizures and almost killed me."[41]

Throughout the House and Senate hearings, members of Congress expressed concerns and raised questions about the health risks associated with ephedra use. U.S. Senator Richard Durbin focused on three issues:

> The obvious questions are these: whether the health concerns announced by Canada and athletic organizations in our own country about ephedra supplements are valid, what actions should be taken by the Department of Health and Human Services and the Food and Drug Administration in light of the Canadian recall, and whether the 1994 law, which Congress enacted, protects American consumers from supplements that may be dangerous to their health."[42]

Meanwhile, dietary supplements containing ephedra had become the most popular weight-loss aids available on the American market. In 2003, the journal *Obesity, Fitness and Wellness Week* estimated that as many as 17 million people were consuming ephedra-based products, gulping down some 3 billion pills a year. The magazine predicted, "The number of consumers that may be injured by this drug could be staggering."[43]

In February 2004 the Food and Drug Administration officially acted, issuing a "final rule" that banned the use of ephedra in all over-the-counter dietary supplements. The FDA, under Commissioner Mark B. McClellan, justified the ephedra ban in a press release, which stated:

> In recent years, dietary supplements containing ephedrine alkaloids have been extensively promoted for aiding weight control and boosting sports performance and energy. The totality of the available data showed little evidence of ephedra's effectiveness except for modest, short-term weight loss without any clear health benefit, while confirming that the substance raises blood pressure and otherwise stresses the circulatory system. These effects are linked to significant adverse health outcomes, including heart attack and stroke.[44]

The ephedra ban went into effect on April 12. However one supplement manufacturer, Nutraceutical Corporation,

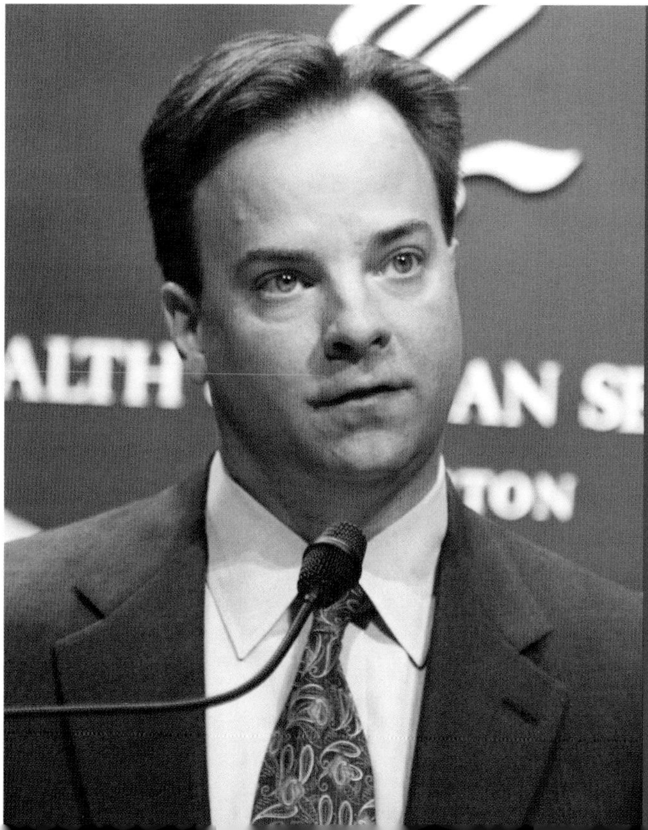

FDA Commissioner Mark B. McClellan notifies consumers and manufacturers that the agency plans to ban the sale and use of the dietary supplement ephedra, December 2003.

A Misplaced Presumption of Safety

Because of the 1994 Dietary Supplement Health and Education Act, the Food and Drug Administration could not ban weight-loss aids containing ephedra—a dietary supplement—without proof that the substance was dangerous. Many people had been under the impression that ephedra-based products were safe simply because they were for sale on store shelves. In fact, according to a 2002 survey, the majority of Americans believe that dietary supplements are regulated by the FDA the same way that prescription drugs and over-the-counter medications are.

In 2002 a market research organization, the Harris Poll, surveyed 1,010 American adults regarding their consumer knowledge of dietary supplements. The results showed that 59 percent believed that the FDA approves dietary supplements for safety and efficacy before they are sold. About 68 percent said that manufacturers have to use warning labels noting potential side effects. Another 55 percent thought the makers of supplement products cannot make claims about product safety without scientific proof. In truth, none of these restrictions exist for dietary supplements.

A former commissioner of the FDA, Dr. Jane E. Henney, told Consumer Reports magazine that when it comes to dietary supplements, "the presumption of safety may have been misplaced, particularly for products other than traditional vitamins and minerals. Some, like ephedra, act like drugs and thus have similar risks."

Quoted in "Dangerous Supplements: Still at Large," *Consumer Reports*, May 2004, www.consumerreports.org/cro/health-fitness/drugs-supplements/dangerous-supplements-504/overview/htm.

which makes products that contain ephedra, sued the FDA because of this action. The following year, in April 2005, federal district court judge Tena Campbell overturned the ban in Utah on the basis that the FDA had not provided sufficient evidence that ephedra at low doses (10 milligrams or less) was dangerous. Many supplement manufacturers saw Campbell's ruling as effectively clearing the way for ephedra to return to store shelves.

Reacting to Campbell's ruling, Kelly Harvey, president of weight-loss supplements distributor TSN Labs, said, "I'm going to spend the rest of the day reading the judge's ruling. Then I'm going to call my manufacturer and give him a new formulation. I'm going to give my label makers a call and order labels. I'm going to be back on the shelves [with ephedra] in five days."[45]

The ruling appalled family members of ephedra victims. Following the death of their son Sean, Debbie and Kevin Riggins had become outspoken critics of the dietary supplements industry. Shortly after Campbell's ruling, Debbie Riggins told the *Peoria Journal Star*, "I can't believe this. I'm surprised one judge can undo this law that so many people worked so hard to get into place to safeguard their kids."[46]

Drastic Steps

Some dietary supplement manufacturers believe the court ruling means they can legally sell products that contain up to 10 milligrams of ephedra. Although the legal position regarding ephedra-based products remains unclear, the FDA continues to consider the substance illegal and has authorized U.S. marshals to seize dietary supplements containing ephedra from their manufacturers.

Many in the weight-loss dietary supplement industry recognize that more information is needed about ephedra before everyone's concerns about the herb are satisfied. In fact, the American Herbal Products Association has recommended to its members that they refrain from marketing ephedra-based supplements until the FDA develops a new set of rules regarding ephedra content. The organization is, however, only a trade association; it has no power to force its members to keep ephedra-based products off store shelves.

Even if products containing small doses of ephedra return to store shelves, their effectiveness remains debatable. Of far greater concern than losing a few pounds of weight should be the health risks associated with the use of any ephedra-based products.

Chapter 5

Drug Abuse and Dieting

It is not only the obese and overweight who take drastic steps to achieve weight loss. People suffering from emotional illnesses that cause eating disorders such as anorexia and bulimia think they are fat even when they actually are painfully thin. In misguided attempts to lose weight, they commonly abuse diuretics, laxatives, or syrup of ipecac. Bodybuilders and other high performance athletes have also turned to drugs such as anabolic steroids in order to change their bodies. In most cases their purpose is not so much to lose weight as to build muscle mass and gain an edge over their competitors. The desire to lose weight has even led some people to take illegal drugs such as methamphetamines, abusing the drugs with little regard to the possible impact on their health.

Anorexia and Bulimia

Maintaining good health often becomes a low priority for people on diets, particularly when they have become dissatisfied with the way they look. Each day, television, film, and print media present images of slender actresses, svelte pop stars, and skinny models dressed in the latest fashions. These celebrities set a standard that few people can meet, although many seek to emulate their examples. Concern with appearances and body image has inspired many people who have perfectly healthy weight to take up the newest diet fads or pick up the latest bottle of diet pills in an effort to trim off some pounds.

Obsession with body image can lead to serious health problems. It is a contributing factor in the development of eating disorders. Traci Mann, a sociologist who has worked with young people with such illnesses, told *People* magazine, "I can tell a girl that what matters is what's going on in her head and heart. But when she turns on the TV, she sees that what matters is how you look."[47]

In people with eating disorders, attempts to diet are taken to extremes. Victims of anorexia nervosa will starve themselves because they are convinced that they are obese—a belief they continue to harbor even as their weight drops to dangerously low levels. They may also engage in high levels of exercise in order to burn up excess calories.

A similar disorder is bulimia nervosa. Like

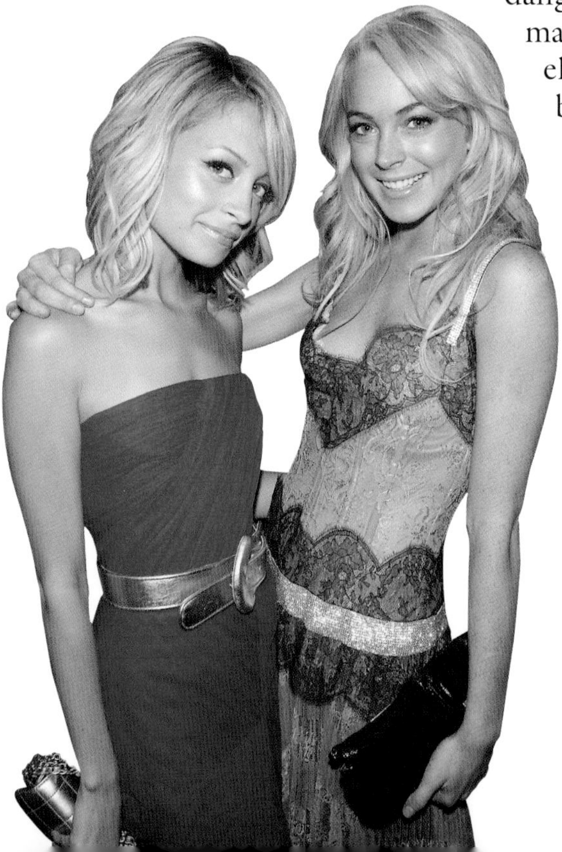

Researchers believe that many women have unhealthy views about their weight because of the media coverage given super-slim celebrities such as actresses Nicole Richie and Lindsay Lohan.

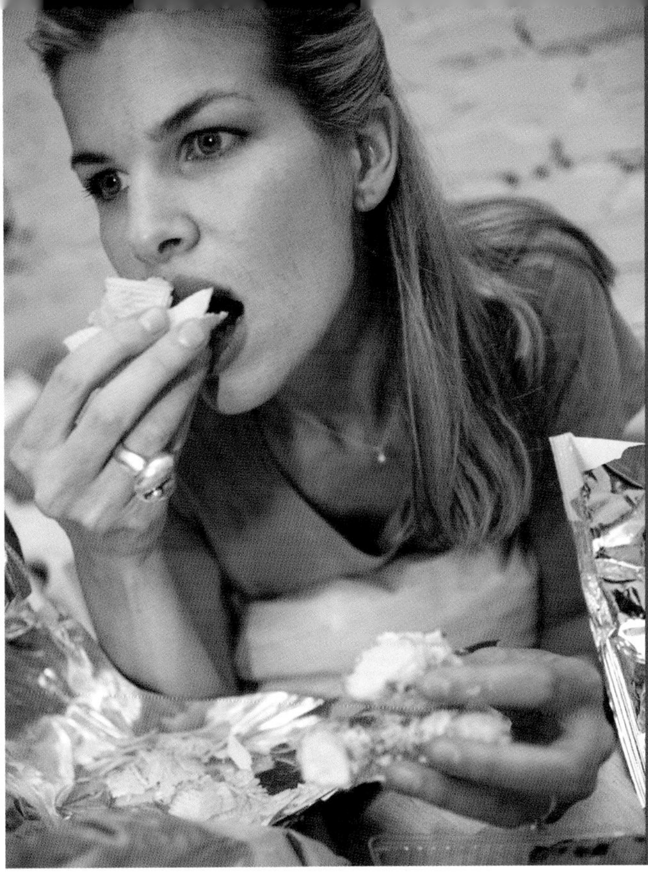

Bulimics go on repeated eating binges, and then purge their bodies of food by taking diuretics, laxatives, or syrup of ipecac.

people with anorexia, bulimics have a distorted body image. They fear that they are obese, but they also suffer from a loss of control when it comes to food. They will go on food binges, or repeated episodes of overeating, and then purge their bodies of food. So that they do not gain weight from binging, they will force themselves to vomit or find other ways to purge.

Anorexia and bulimia primarily affect teenage girls and women in their early twenties. However, researchers believe that as many as one in ten anorexics and bulimics are boys and young men. In recent years, more women in their thirties, forties, and fifties have been diagnosed as anorexic and bulimic. "These days, you have to be young and gorgeous, even at 50,"[48] says Dr. Holly Grishkat, a supervisor at a Philadelphia eating disorders clinic. Regardless of gender and age, it is not unusual for bulimics as well as anorexics to turn to drugs to lose weight.

Risky Weight-Loss Techniques

A poll conducted by *People* magazine in 2000 found that some women practice risky behavior when trying to lose weight. The poll, which queried a thousand women, said that 5 percent have tried laxatives to lose weight, while another 5 percent said they purge their bodies through vomiting. As many as 23 percent said they have tried fasting, while 12 percent said they have smoked cigarettes as a way of killing their appetites. Another 35 percent said they have tried over-the-counter diet pills, while 16 percent have turned to prescription diet pills.

The majority of woman, however, indicated that they follow good weight-loss programs of exercising (86.5 percent), dieting (72 percent), and eating smaller portions (60 percent). A small proportion of respondents said they have resorted to alternative practices to lose weight such as hypnosis (4 percent) and acupuncture (3 percent). Only 1 percent used surgery to lose weight.

Christy's Story

The story of Christy Henrich provides a tragic example of what eating disorders can do. In 1988, at the age of sixteen, she just missed making the cut for the U.S. Olympic women's gymnastic team. Henrich immediately set her sights on winning a spot on the team for the 1992 games, and began to train harder. A year later, it appeared that she was on the right track. In 1989, she placed second overall in the U.S. championships and fourth on the uneven parallel bars in the world championships.

Henrich weighed 90 pounds (40.8kg) in 1988, but after a gymnastics judge told the four-foot, ten-inch girl she would have a better chance of reaching the Olympics if she lost weight, Henrich became obsessed with the idea of shedding pounds. It was an obsession that would cost Henrich her health, her career, and ultimately her life.

In her efforts to lose weight, Henrich maintained a rigorous regimen of training each day for six or seven hours, and she subsisted on very little food. At one point, she ate just an apple a day, a diet later reduced to only a slice of an apple per day. Like most anorexics, Henrich denied that she had an eating disorder. By the time friends and family members forced her to seek help, she had lost 27 pounds (12.2kg), and weighed a mere 63 pounds (28.6kg).

In 1992, the year Henrich had hoped to be competing at the U.S. Olympics, she was instead checking into a clinic in Topeka, Kansas, for treatment for anorexia. Her boyfriend, Bo Moreno, told *Sports Illustrated* that he warned Henrich's parents to check her suitcase carefully as they unpacked her belongings at the clinic. "It had a false bottom," he said. "She had lined the entire bottom of the suitcase with laxatives. That was part of her addiction."[49]

Using Laxatives to Purge

Laxatives are one method used by anorexics and bulimics to purge their bodies of food. They are available in supermarkets and pharmacies without prescription, and can range from mild to powerful.

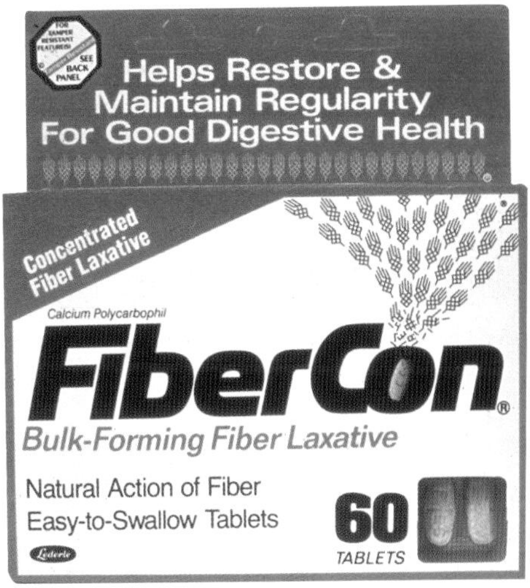

Bulimics commonly use laxatives in the erroneous belief that they purge the body of food before it can be digested and cause weight gain.

Anorexics and bulimics commonly use laxatives in the belief that these drugs force food through the gastrointestinal system before it can be fully digested and metabolized into fat. However, that is a myth. Laxatives work toward the end of the bowel, after the nutrients in food have already been absorbed into the body.

Overuse of laxatives can lead to serious health problems. These drugs purge the body of fluids and cause dehydration, a potentially life-threatening condition. Long-term use of laxatives can also remove important minerals such as potassium, magnesium, sodium, and chloride—elements that the body needs to function properly.

Christy Henrich fought her illness for several years, but the cycles of starvation and purging destroyed her health. Just before she died—at the age of twenty-two—Henrich slipped into a coma. "She was getting intensive supportive care," stated her doctor, David McKinsey. "But a person passes the point of no return, and then, no matter how aggressive the care is, it doesn't work. The major problem is a severe lack of fuel. The person becomes so malnourished that the liver doesn't work, the kidneys don't work, and neither do the muscles. The cells no longer function."[50]

Other Drugs Used for Weight Loss

People with eating disorders may also try to lose weight by taking diuretics, or water pills. These drugs remove fluid and salts in the body by inducing urination. Some of the familiar brands include Aqua-Ban, Diurex, and Watertix Plus. High school and college wrestlers looking to lose a few pounds before a match so they can qualify for their desired weight class have been known to abuse such products. However, like laxatives, water pills do not rid the body of fat. The drugs produce a temporary and minor weight loss.

Anorexics and bulimics may also purge by inducing vomiting with a drug called syrup of ipecac. This product, which has been available for years as an over-the-counter medication, is

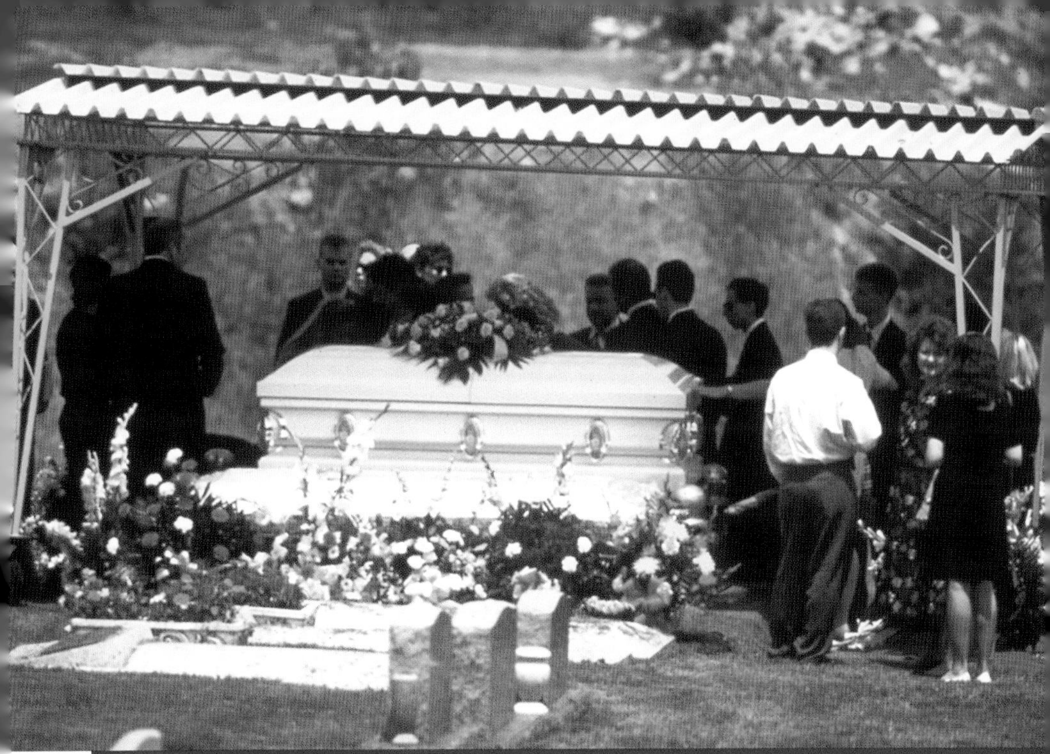

Family and friends attend the 1994 funeral of gymnast Christy Henrich. During her struggle with anorexia nervosa and bulimia, Henrich abused laxatives to lose weight.

used to induce vomiting in victims of accidental poisonings. Before the introduction of child-proof caps on prescription bottles, household cleaners, and other toxic substances, most families kept a bottle of ipecac in the medicine cabinet in case a young child ingested a poisonous substance.

Health Consequences

Forcing oneself to vomit, either with or without drugs, carries health risks. The bulimic cycle of binging and purging can damage the digestive tract by causing bleeding in the esophagus—the tube that carries food to the stomach. The ongoing cycle of purging by vomiting can also cause chemical imbalances in the body that damage the heart, resulting in irregular heartbeat, heart failure, and death. During the act of vomiting, fluid can enter the respiratory tract, causing gagging or even choking. As with laxatives and diuretics, excessive vomiting can also lead to dehydration.

Anorexia is a particularly deadly disease because it involves starving the body. Anorexics often suffer serious complications from malnutrition, the deficiency in nutrients (vitamins, minerals, and other substances) the body needs to function normally. With fewer calories to burn, the body slows down in an effort to conserve the energy it has. The result is an abnormally slow heart rate and low blood pressure, which impairs the heart muscle and increases the risk of heart failure.

As the weight falls to dangerously low levels, females stop producing the hormone estrogen and stop menstruating. Low estrogen levels lead to losses in bone density, which makes the bones brittle and susceptible to breakage, a condition known as osteoporosis. Muscle loss may cause cardiac arrest, or dehydration may cause the body's liver, kidneys, and other organs shut down.

A Difficult Struggle

The life-threatening eating disorders of anorexia and bulimia affect an estimated 10 million women and 1.1 million men in the United States. These illnesses strike not only those aspiring to be like celebrities, but also the famous as well. In the summer of 2004, just before turning age 18, the actress Mary-Kate Olsen checked into an eating disorder center for six weeks to treat anorexia. Other celebrities who have admitted to having eating disorders include actress Christina Ricci, pop singer and *American Idol* judge Paula Abdul, and actor Billy Bob Thornton.

Bulimia survivor and television actress Jamie-Lynn DiScala authored an autobiography, entitled *Wise Girl*, in which she recounted her personal experiences with the eating disorder. In addition to writing about her illness, DiScala also serves as a spokesperson for the National Eating Disorder Association, a nonprofit organization that helps people dealing with anorexia, bulimia, and binge eating disorders.

While actors and actresses develop eating disorders because of the goal to look good, many athletes become anorexic and

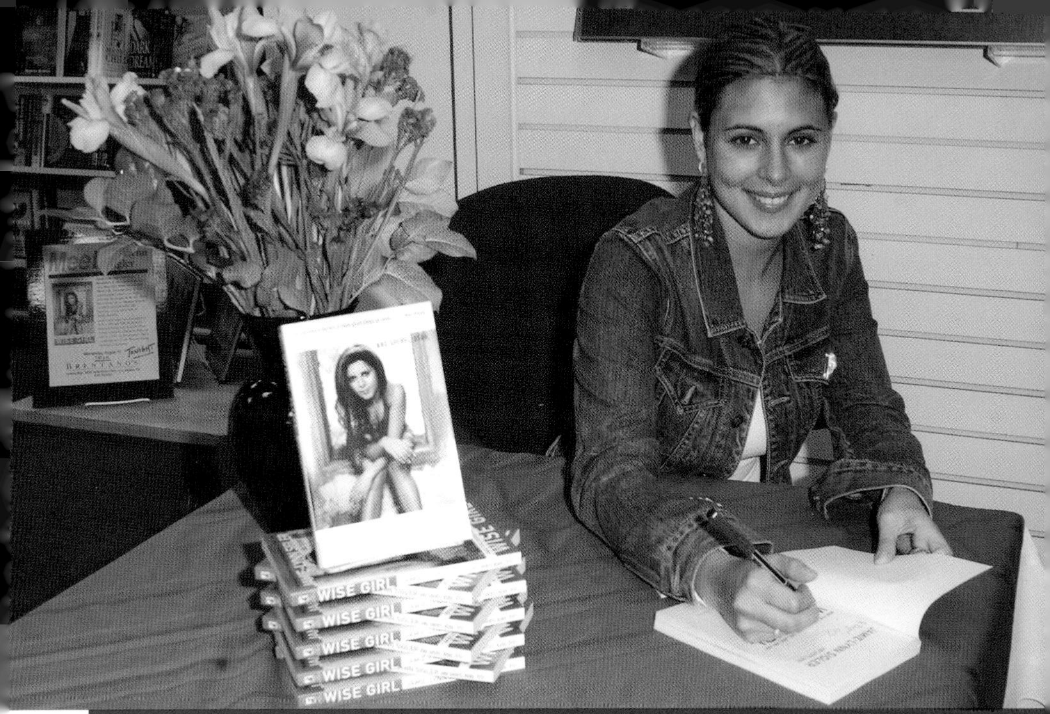

Actor Jamie-Lynn DiScala wrote a book about her battle with bulimia. She currently serves as a spokesperson for National Eating Disorders Association.

bulimic because of their sport. The potential to develop eating disorders is particularly high among those participating in gymnastics, diving, bodybuilding, and wrestling—sports in which participants must meet weight or size requirements. But such pressures can occur in all high-level sports. For example, more than one third of the young women participating in a study of Division 1 NCAA athletes reported attitudes and symptoms that placed them at risk for anorexia nervosa.

Steroid Abuse

The desire to achieve peak performance in sports can lead to the abuse of another kind of drug—anabolic steroids. Many high-performance athletes, bodybuilders, and weightlifters looking to build up muscle mass and reduce body fat have turned to steroids, which are synthetically made substances related to the male sex hormones.

Although legally available only by prescription, anabolic steroids have found their way into the hands of people of all ages, including middle and high school athletes and professional sports players. In 2005 a series of congressional hearings on steroid use in professional sports focused on the popularity of these drugs among many baseball players. The same year, a study by the sports medicine division of Oregon Health and Science University reported an increase in steroid use among teenage girls. Researchers concluded that the girls are not seeking an edge on the playing field but rather are trying to sculpt their bodies in the images of models and movie stars. "With young women, you see them using it more as a weight control and body fat reduction"[51] method, said Rutgers University counselor Jeff Hoerger.

Syrup of Ipecac

Syrup of ipecac is extracted from the root of ipecacuanha, a small shrubby plant that grows in South America, mostly in Brazil. The plant's ability to induce vomiting was well known to South American Indians at the time Portuguese explorers arrived on the continent during the early 1500s. The Europeans named the plant *ipecacuanha*, after the native word *i-pe-kaa-guéne*, which is said to mean "roadside sick-making plant."

Ipecac contains large quantities of the chemical emetine, which causes vomiting. In fact, the English word *emetic* means to induce vomiting. However, when administered in very small doses, ipecac can ease the stomach and intestines, helping digestion and stimulating appetite—quite the opposite effect desired by bulimics and anorexics using the drug.

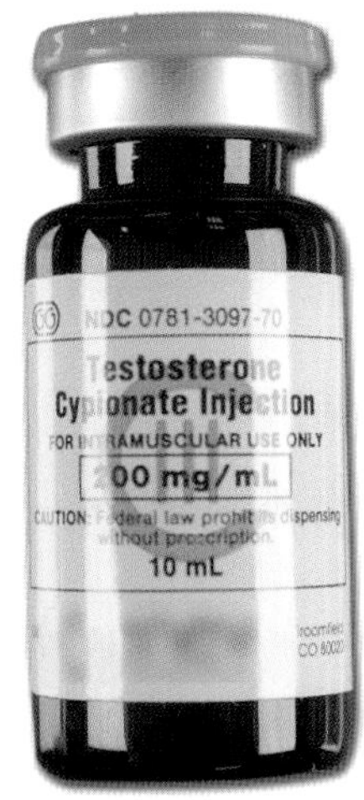

Some young women have used steroids to help them lose weight. However, these drugs can cause serious side effects.

Steroid abuse can lead to many long-lasting and potentially fatal consequences. Once in the body, steroids are converted into the male hormone testosterone, which helps the body process protein into muscle mass. The typical male body produces about ten milligrams of testosterone a day. People who abuse steroids often consume doses that help them produce hundreds of milligrams.

By stimulating such massive amounts of testosterone, people taking the drug to sculpt their bodies can expect to see results within weeks, but they will also start experiencing side effects as well. Boys and men often find that their bodies stop producing their own testosterone. The glands that produce testosterone—the testes—start shrinking and eventually may lose the ability to produce the hormone. Because the testes also produce sperm, steroid use may lower sperm count and cause infertility in males. Girls and women who take steroids may lose their hair; grow hair on the face, back, and chest; and experience irregular menstrual cycles.

Other adverse effects of steroid use include bloating, blood-clotting disorders, liver damage, heart attacks and stroke, high blood pressure, kidney problems, and cancer. Steroids can also be addictive, and their abuse can cause psychological problems, such as fits of anger known as "roid rage" and other irrational behavior.

Methamphetamine

Similar psychological behaviors of rage and irrationality have occurred in people using the illegal drug methamphetamine, or meth, as a diet drug. A form of amphetamine, meth stimulates the central nervous system, creating a sense of alertness and euphoria in the user. The drug is mostly manufactured illegally in meth laboratories using ephedrine and pseudoephedrine (an ingredient found in many over-the-counter drugs).

During the 1950s and 1960s, methamphetamine was marketed as the diet drug Desoxyn, but in 1970 it was classified as a Schedule II drug under the Controlled Substances Act. Although most people take meth today as a recreational drug—for its mood enhancing qualities—increasing numbers of people are obtaining the drug illegally for the purpose of losing weight. Its users report that the drug suppresses the appetite and allows them to lose weight very quickly.

However, the people taking methamphetamine for weight control are ignoring the serious health risks that accompany the use of this illegal drug. Because the stimulant produces such a strong effect on the central nervous system, it is highly addictive. Other serious adverse effects caused by the powerful stimulant include psychotic episodes and heart and neuro-

Although Desoxyn, a form of methamphetamine, is occasionally prescribed for weight loss, most users acquire the drug illegally. Chunks of crystal meth are pictured below, while two Desoxyn tablets are shown in the inset.

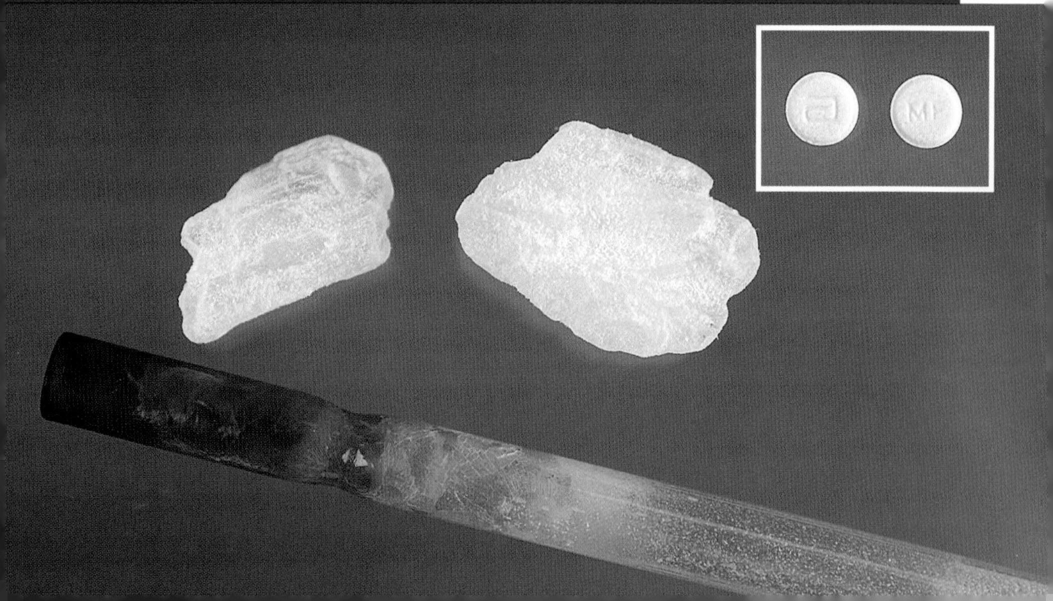

logical damage. People taking meth are prone to violent and aggressive actions, and many suffer from memory loss after long-term use. Despite the serious problems that occur with meth abuse, some women continue to risk their health—and potentially their lives—by taking the illicit drug simply to lose weight.

Making Healthy Choices

Abusing drugs to achieve weight loss may provide the desired results, but often at great risk to a person's overall health. While few people looking to drop a few pounds would go to such extremes as drug abuse, many think nothing of occasionally swallowing diet drugs or weight-loss supplements. In search of an easy way to lose weight, they overlook the potential for adverse effects that comes with taking any medication or supplement.

Most physicians prefer to guide patients through weight-loss programs that do not depend on the use of diet drugs, but focus instead on healthy lifestyle habits that include eating a low-calorie, nutritional diet and exercising regularly. When used under a doctor's guidance, certain diet drugs can effectively kick-start a severely obese patient's program to lose weight. For most everyone else, though, healthy lifestyle choices remain the most effective way to slim down and keep the weight off.

NOTES

Introduction: Diet Drugs: No Miracle Cures

1. Quoted in U.S. Senate Committee on Governmental Affairs, *Hearings on When Diets Turn Deadly: Consumer Safety and Weight-Loss Supplements*, July 31, 2002.

Chapter 1: A History of Dieting and Drug Use

2. Quoted in Adelaide Hechtlinger, *The Great Patent Medicine Era*. New York: Galahad Books, 1970, p. 37.
3. Quoted in Hechtlinger, *The Great Patent Medicine Era*, p. 231.
4. Quoted in Hechtlinger, *The Great Patent Medicine Era*, p. 231.
5. Quoted in Edward M. Brecher, *Licit and Illicit Drugs*. Mount Vernon, NY: Consumers Union, 1972, p. 296.
6. Jim Bouton, *Ball Four*. New York: Dell Publishing, 1970, p. 80.
7. Bouton, *Ball Four*, p. 159.
8. Quoted in Matthew Heller, "Death and Denial at Herbalife: The Untold Story of Mark Hughes' Public Image, Secret Vice and Tragic Destiny," *Los Angeles Times Magazine*, February 18, 2001, p. 12.

Chapter 2: The Fen-Phen Debacle

9. Quoted in Michael D. Lemonick, "Health: The New Miracle Drug?" *Time*, September 23, 1996, p. 61.
10. Quoted in Lemonick, "Health: The New Miracle Drug?" p. 61.
11. Quoted in David Stipp, "New Weapons in the War on Fat," *Fortune*, December 11, 1995, p. 164.
12. Quoted in Lemonick, "Health: The New Miracle Drug?" p. 61.

13. Quoted in Lemonick, "Health: The New Miracle Drug?" p. 61.
14. Quoted in *PBS Frontline*, "Dangerous Prescription," November 13, 2003. www.pbs.org/wgbh/pages/frontline/shows/prescription/interviews/rich.html.
15. Quoted in Alicia Mundy, *Dispensing with the Truth: The Victims, the Drug Companies, and the Dramatic Story Behind the Battle over Fen-Phen.* New York: St. Martin's Press, 2001, p. 283.
16. Quoted in CBS News, "Diet Pill May Help Obese Teens," June 15, 2005. www.cbsnews.com/stories/2005/06/15/earlyshow/health/health_news/main702018.shtml
17. Quoted in CBS News, "Diet Pill May Help Obese Teens."
18. Quoted in Shari Roan, "Diet Drug May Go over the Counter," *Los Angeles Times*, October 24, 2005. www.latimes.com/features/health/nutrition/la-he-obesity24oct24,1,546146.story?coll=la-health-nutrition-news

Chapter 3: Weight-loss Dietary Supplements

19. Dexatrim Dietary Supplements. "Dexatrim Results," www.dexatrim.com/product_results.asp
20. Anna Nicole Smith, "How I Lost More than 60 Pounds!" *Us*, March 1, 2004, p. 48.
21. Bennett Alan Weinberg and Bonnie K. Bealer, *The Caffeine Advantage.* New York: Free Press, 2002, p. 161.
22. Weinberg and Bealer, *The Caffeine Advantage*, pp.160–161.
23. *Tufts University Health & Nutrition Letter*, "Green Tea for Weight Loss?" June 1, 2003, p. 3.
24. Quoted in *CNN Daybreak*, "What's the Deal with Some of the Newer Weight Loss Supplements?" November 12, 2003. http://transcripts.cnn.com/TRANSCRIPTS/0311/12/lad.14.html
25. Quoted in Mary Duenwald, "An Appetite Killer for a Killer Appetite? Not Yet," *New York Times*, April 19, 2005, p. 5-5.

26. Robert B. Saper, David M. Eisenberg, and Russell S. Phillips, "Common Dietary Supplements for Weight Loss," *American Family Physician*, Nov. 1, 2004, pp. 1,731–1,732.
27. Saper, Eisenberg, and Phillips, "Common Dietary Supplements for Weight Loss," p. 1,735.
28. American Herbal Products Association, "Herbal FAQs: Are Herbal Supplement Products Safe?" www.ahpa.org/herbal_faqs.htm.
29. Quoted in *NPR Talk of the Nation*, "Safety and Regulation of Dietary Supplements," November 1, 2000.
30. Congresswoman Susan A. Davis, "Floor Statement: Dietary Supplement Access and Awareness Act," June 30, 2005. www.house.gov/susandavis/statements/st063005dsaa.html

Chapter 4: Ephedra and Its Dangers

31. Quoted in Shannon Brownlee, "Swallowing Ephedra," Salon.com, June 7, 2000. www.salon.com/health/feature/2000/06/07/ephedra/index.html
32. Quoted in *NPR All Things Considered*, "Profile: Politics and Lobbying in the U.S. Nutritional and Dietary Supplements Industry," June 23, 2003.
33. Quoted in *CNN American Morning with Paula Zahn*, "Interview with Bechler Family Attorney," February 27, 2003. http://transcripts.cnn.com/TRANSCRIPTS/0302/27/ltm.12.html
34. Quoted in L. Jon Wertheim, "Jolt of Reality: Following the Lead of Elite Athletes, Teenagers Are Increasingly Juicing Their Workouts with Pills and Powders—Sometimes with Tragic Results," *Sports Illustrated*, April 7, 2003, p. 68.
35. Quoted in Wertheim, "Jolt of Reality," p. 68.
36. Quoted in Mike Fillon, *Ephedra: Fact & Fiction*. Orem, Utah: Woodland Publishing, 2003, p. 116.
37. Quoted in Fillon, *Ephedra: Fact & Fiction*, p. 118.
38. Quoted in Fillon, *Ephedra: Fact & Fiction*, p. 118.
39. Quoted in Amanda Spake, "Natural Hazards," *U.S. News and World Report*, February 12, 2001, pp. 43–49.

40. U.S. Senate Committee on Commerce, Science and Transportation, *Hearings on Dangers of Dietary Supplements*, October 28, 2003, p. 30.
41. Senate Committee, *Hearings on Dangers of Dietary Supplements*, p. 31.
42. Quoted in U.S. Senate Committee on Governmental Affairs, *Hearings on When Diets Turn Deadly: Consumer Safety and Weight Loss Supplements.* July 31, 2002, p. 3.
43. Business & Industry Database. "Dietary Supplements: More Deaths Related to Ephedra Products," *Obesity, Fitness & Wellness Week*, April 26, 2003, p. 15.
44. U.S. Food and Drug Administration, "FDA Issues Regulation Prohibiting Sale of Dietary Supplements Containing Ephedrine Alkaloids and Reiterates Its Advice That Consumers Stop Using These Products," Feb. 6, 2004. www.cfsan.fda.gov/~lrd/fpephed6.html
45. Quoted in "Ephedra Ban Lifted by Judge in Utah," *Salt Lake Tribune*, April 15, 2005.
46. Quoted in Jessica L. Aberle, "Judge Strikes Ephedra Ban—Federal Case Upsets Lincoln Family Whose Son's Death Was Linked to Supplement," *Peoria Journal Star*, April 15, 2005.

Chapter 5: Drug Abuse and Dieting

47. Quoted in Kim Hubbard, Anne-Marie O'Neill, and Christina Cheakalos, "Out of Control: Weight-Obsessed, Stressed-Out Coeds Are Increasingly Falling Prey to Eating Disorders," *People*, April 12, 1999, p. 52.
48. Quoted in Ericka Sóuter et al. "Adult Anorexia: Once Primarily a Teen Affliction, Eating Disorders Are Affecting Women in Their 30s and Beyond," *People*, June 6, 2005, pp. 87–88.
49. Quoted in Merrell Noden, "Dying to Win," *Sports Illustrated*, August 8, 1994, p. 52.
50. Quoted in Noden, "Dying to Win," p. 52.
51. Quoted in Linda A. Johnson, "Steroid Use on Rise Among Girls," Associated Press, April 26, 2005.

Organizations to Contact

American Herbal Products Association
8484 Georgia Avenue
Suite 370
Silver Spring, MD 20910
(301) 588-1171
Web site: www.ahpa.org

The American Herbal Products Association is a trade organization that represents the manufacturers of dietary supplements and acts as an advocate for the industry during congressional hearings and similar forums. Visitors to the organization's Web site can find press releases and answers to frequently asked questions about herbal supplements.

American Obesity Association (ABO)
1250 24th Street, NW
Suite 300
Washington, DC 20037
(202) 776-7711
Web site: www.obesity.org

The organization takes the position that obesity is a disease and supports efforts to provide public education about the dangers of obesity. The American Obesity Association has pressured the Food and Drug Administration to closely monitor companies that manufacture weight loss supplements. The organization's Web site contains a "Consumer Alert" link that alerts dieters to the dangers of dietary supplements.

Center for Science in the Public Interest (CSPA)
1875 Connecticut Ave. N.W.
Suite 300
Washington, DC 20009
(202) 332-9110
Web site: www.cspinet.org

The consumerism group advocates for strict governmental regulation over the dietary supplements industry. CSPA also takes positions and provides research papers on a number of other food and nutrition-related topics, including mad cow disease, food additives, genetic engineering of crops, and snack food sales in schools.

U.S. Centers for Disease Control and Prevention
1600 Clifton Road
Atlanta, GA 30333
(800) 311-3435
Web site: www.cdc.gov

The federal government's chief public health agency has performed many studies on obesity, which can be accessed at the agency's Web site.

U.S. Federal Trade Commission (FTC)
600 Pennsylvania Avenue NW
Washington, DC 20580
877 382-4357
Web site: www.ftc.gov

The federal agency charged with ensuring truth in advertising has conducted a number of studies on how weight-loss supplements are marketed. The reports can be accessed at the FTC's Web site by following the link for "Diet and Fitness."

U. S. Food and Drug Administration (FDA)
5600 Fishers Lane
Rockville MD 20857-0001
(888) 463-6332
Web site: www.fda.gov

Periodicals

Sally Squires, "Pills for Losers: American's Hunger for Diet-Aid Supplements Outweighs Unknowns." *Washington Post*, December 13, 2005. Overview of Americans' use of weight-loss dietary supplements.

L. John Wertheim, "Jolt of Reality: Following the Lead of Elite Athletes, Teenagers Are Increasingly Juicing Their Workouts with Pills and Powders—Sometimes with Tragic Results," *Sports Illustrated*, April 7, 2003. The magazine article traces the story of Sean Riggins, the Illinois high school athlete who died after consuming ephedra-based diet pills.

Internet Sources

PBS Frontline, "Dangerous Prescription." www.pbs.org/wgbh/pages/frontline/shows/prescription. Companion Web site to the *PBS Frontline* documentary on the effectiveness of the Food and Drug Administration in protecting Americans from dangerous drugs. Includes an overview of fen-phen approval as a prescription drug by the FDA and the consequences.

U.S. Centers for Disease Control, "Overweight and Obesity." www.cdc.gov/nccdphp/dnpa/obesity. This page provides official government statistics on obesity, as well as links to reports on the problem.

INDEX

Picture Credits

Cover: © Corbis
AP/Wide World Photos, 63, 64, 71
© Brian Bailey/Corbis, 68
© Bettmann/Corbis, 17
Stephen Chernin/Getty Images, 38
Getty Images, 78
© Gianni Dagli Orti/Corbis, 14
Steve Kagan/Time Life Pictures/Getty Images, 35
Robert King/Newsmakers/Getty Images, 44
© Marvin Koner/Corbis, 25
© Michelle Lawlor, 11, 51, 55
Buck Miller/Time Life Pictures/Getty Images, 83
Robert Mora/Getty Images, 85
Ralph Notaro/Getty Images, 48
© OTTN Publishing, 10, 28, 36
PhotoDisc, 79
Joe Raedle/Getty Images, 9, 41
Mario Ruiz/Time Life Pictures/Getty Images, 81
© Swim Ink 2, LLC/Corbis, 21
Allan Tannenbaum/Time Life Pictures/Getty Images, 31
Time Life Pictures/Getty Images, 32
U.S. Drug Enforcement Administration, 40, 87, 88
Courtesy of Utah Museum of Natural History, Garrett Herbarium, 60
Mark Wilson/Getty Images, 73
Alex Wong/Getty Images, 52

About the Author

Hal Marcovitz is a journalist who lives in Chalfont, Pennsylvania, with his wife Gail and daughters Michelle and Ashley. He has written more than seventy books for young readers as well as the satirical novel *Painting the White House*.